Everything You've Always Wanted To Know About Cannabis But Were Afraid To Ask

It's Not Just for Stoners

D. Marie Dumas

Table of Contents

Dedication

This book is dedicated to all those seeking the truth as it relates to cannabis, to patients battling various illnesses and searching for natural and/or alternative methods and nutraceuticals, and to all those that have suffered more harm than good by prescribed medications (pharmaceuticals).

Acknowledgments

I would like to first thank my family and dearest friends for their deep love and support during my battle with breast cancer. Especially my father, J. L. Dumas, and my sister, Jolika Dumas. To say that they were my "rock" would be a gross understatement!

I also want to thank my "gang", specifically Roy McCloud and Jill Anderson, I could not possibly have asked for greater friends! Their love, support, prayers, and faith were deeply appreciated, even when I didn't ask – I knew they were praying for me!

Lastly, I would like to thank my physician, Dr. Mark Hertzberg whose zest for life, encouragement, and humor helped me in my efforts to remain positive and hopeful – not to mention the various nutraceutical supplements he recommended that did my body only good!

To all the physicians, scientists, research teams, and herbalists for sharing their discoveries to date in their endeavor to make known the benefits (as well as the cautions) relating to cannabis use. I say with heartfelt gratitude – THANK YOU!

About The Author

Marie Dumas is a breast cancer survivor; having to battle cancer and the negative side effects experienced by prescribed pharmaceuticals set her on a path to research natural remedies for cancer and various illnesses, whether it is something as simple as the common cold or something as potentially life-threatening as cancer. Her goal is to be one of the vehicles to help rid society of the negative stereotypes associated with cannabis use.

Author's Note

One of my intentions for writing this book is to help remove the stigma and negative stereotypes associated with the consumption of cannabis/marijuana. With this in mind, I will leave it to the reader to explore what I have managed to assemble, such as learning how much marijuana can help decrease the risk of some cancers, how much it helps cancer patients reduce the pain and side effects after going through chemotherapy, radiation, and other forms of treatment, as well as many other ailments in which cannabis consumption has helped countless patients overcome.

Although I am not a marijuana smoker, I have taken a great deal of time to compile many of the benefits that marijuana can bring to one's life in general. From my studies, I have discovered that properly consuming marijuana can help with various ailments without the negative side effects that many pharmaceuticals/synthetic drugs have been known to cause. While some can argue that the results are largely short-term, the experience of countless patients has proven real and lasting results.

Over the past few decades, we have experienced increased usage of marijuana, both for social consumption and medicinal purposes. Nevertheless, despite the positive strides made in legalizing marijuana consumption, we are still experiencing equal amounts of resistance by our current government, as they erroneously deem this substance dangerous and thus still illegal in many places.

It is my desire that you gain useful, helpful information from this book; I prepared it not as an encouragement to simply "get high", but to be responsible with consumption in order to keep us healthy, both physically and mentally.

Be informed, be blessed, and be healed.

D. Marie Dumas

Disclaimer

This book is not exhaustive on the subject of cannabis, nor is it intended as a substitute for the medical advice of physicians. The reader should regularly consult a physician in matters relating to his/her health and particularly with respect to any symptoms that may require diagnosis and/or medical attention.

 References in the book are provided solely for informational purposes and do not constitute endorsement of any agencies, institutions, or websites.

Foreword

"Marijuana is a medicine. Marijuana is NOT a drug."

- Dr. Sebi

Ms. D. Dumas has written a very timely and relevant book on the positive and healing virtues of marijuana. This book is absolutely needed now, especially in the African-American community, where blacks have historically been victims of racist drug laws. She is following the same path as sacred science health advocates, like the late great Dr. Sebi. Dr. Sebi was an African herbalist, dietitian, and holistic health specialist. He was born Alfredo Darrington Bowman in Honduras in 1933.

In an interview from Honduras, Sebi stated that 'weed' is actually a natural healing medicine plant. He states, "As far as the issue of marijuana is concerned, there should be no issue," he said. "If it is an issue, then all other herbs that are natural should be an issue. Marijuana is a sacred and natural plant. It comes from the family of the carbon chain. It is known in genecology as a native plant from the lily of the valley. I recommend it. I thank God for having produced it because it helped me with my asthma as a child. I am willing to debate with the top scientists in the U.S. about how and why marijuana is not harmful as a natural plant," Sebi said.

Congresswoman Suzanne Bonamici (D-Ore.) introduced legislation to legalize the use of marijuana nationally. She stated, "My bipartisan amendment is very simple. It would move our country in line with industrialized countries around the world that long ago recognized the importance of industrial hemp as a natural resource, an agricultural commodity, and a versatile component in thousands of commercial products," Bonamici said at the hearing.

The war on marijuana is racist. That's the conclusion of a major report (06/04/2013) by the American Civil Liberties Union (ACLU). Among the alarming findings in "The War on Marijuana in Black & White" is that while marijuana use rates between blacks and whites are comparable, blacks are nearly four times more likely to be arrested for marijuana possession.

The report – the first to evaluate marijuana arrests rates by race on a national scope – finds that the disparity isn't just limited to inner cities. In over 96 percent of the counties the ACLU examined, which cover 78 percent of the U.S. population, blacks are arrested at higher rates than whites for marijuana possession. And, while criminal justice observers have long known that drug arrests are conducted on a racially disproportionate basis, the report finds that the disparity has widened even further over the past decade. ACLU's analysis reveals that while annual marijuana arrests have risen over 10 years, the arrest rate for whites remained constant, meaning that the overall national increase in arrests is largely attributable to a whole lot more black people getting busted.

This clear unfair targeting of our nation's failed marijuana laws has prompted a growing number of leaders from black communities to raise their voices in favor of reform. Several state branches of the NAACP have endorsed legalization and played a crucial role in last year's successful campaigns to end marijuana prohibition in Colorado and Washington State. Mayor Cory Booker of Newark, NJ, has declared war on drugs a failure and endorsed reforms like medical marijuana laws. Jesse Jackson called the drug war "a new Jim Crow offensive against people of color." Al Sharpton says racial disparities in drug law enforcement have "undermined the legitimacy of our criminal justice system." And Actor Morgan Freeman says marijuana prohibition is "just the stupidest law possible."

Thank you, Ms. Dumas, for this game-changing book.

- Michael Moss Ph.D., author of "Sankofa Sacred Science."

Preface

The purpose of this book is two-fold: As previously mentioned, this publication is intended to educate the public about cannabis with the hopes of aiding in the removal of the negative stigma and stereotypes associated with it, and secondly, but most importantly, to share the many valuable medical benefits that marijuana has provided (and is still providing) to patients with various illnesses and conditions. There exists quite a bit of negative propaganda surrounding cannabis use, not to mention the misinformation purported by government entities. Nevertheless, I am dedicated to helping dispel the myths by sharing some of the many ways that cannabis use can help rather than hurt individuals and the world at large. As the author, I hope that this book will aid the reader in understanding the beneficial aspects and the multi-layered components of cannabis/marijuana.

1. Introduction

What Exactly Is Marijuana?

Marijuana has been known by various nicknames throughout the years. Amongst those names, it is most commonly known as weed, pot, ganja, Mary Jane, hemp, and cannabis, to name a few. Marijuana is the female flower bud of the plant Cannabis sativa, Cannabis indica, or a hybrid of both strains. The male flower buds have very minimal psychedelic properties, if any at all, and therefore are not as psychoactive as the female flower. Of the 483 known compounds in the plant, there are 86 cannabinoid chemicals identified. Of those 86 chemicals, the main psychoactive chemical in marijuana is called *tetrahydrocannabinol* (THC). Some of the other cannabinoid chemicals found are *cannabidiol* (CBD), *cannabinol* (CBN), *tetrahydrocannabinol acid (THCA), cannabaravin* (THCV), *cannabichromene* (CBC), *cannabigerol* (CBG), and *cannbicyclol* (CBL); these terms along with others will be defined later in subsequent chapters.

All of these cannabinoid chemicals are known to also have psychoactive and pharmacological properties. Since THC and CBD are the chemicals in which most marijuana users are interested, the herb's potency is typically measured in THC and CBD concentrations. Although these chemicals are found in the whole plant (less than 0.5% for inactive hemp and 2 to 3% for marijuana leaves), the female cannabis flower bud glands (4 to 20% concentration) is where the chemicals are the strongest and provide the most psychoactive, euphoric effect.

What is interesting about the cannabinoids is that their high lipid-soluble ability (this refers to the power of a substance dissolving into lipids, fats, and oils), they can stay within the body for an extended amount of time. Even though the THC is broken down in the liver to THC-COOH (the chemical that urine tests detect), the chemical can stay within the body for four days for occasional users and 67 days for extreme or chronic users. Numerous researchers have suggested that perhaps this special ability allows cannabis to effectively treat so many different health problems since it can readily be absorbed into the lipid membranes of neurons and other cells within the body.

1.1 Our Body's Endocannabinoid System

Most of us are aware or have heard of the human body's various systems such as the central nervous system, the digestive system, the circulatory system, the endocrine system, etc.. Still, very few are aware of the *Endogenous Cannabinoid System (ECS),* which was named after the plant that led to its discovery. Endogenous means "*produced or synthesized within the organism or system", or more simply put, endo means "within" and genous means "arising from"... thus arising from within.*

The endocannabinoid system is a bridge between the body and the mind and is probably the most important physiologic system involved in establishing and maintaining our health. Endocannabinoids and their receptors are found all throughout our body, in the brain, organs, connective tissues, glands, and immune cells. In each of these areas, the cannabinoid system performs different tasks, but the goal is always the same for each area – *homeostasis*, which is the maintenance of a stable internal environment, regardless of changes in the external environment.

Cannabinoids promote a stable environment at every level of biological life – from the organism to the sub-cellular. One example of this is a process called *autophagy*, which is the body's way of cleaning out damaged cells in order to create newer, healthier cells. This process is enabled by the cannabinoid system. It keeps normal/healthy cells alive and has a deadly effect on malignant tumor cells, causing them to consume themselves in a programmed cellular suicide (*apoptosis*). Naturally, the death of cancer cells promotes homeostasis and survival at the level of the entire organism.

Endocannabinoids and cannabinoids are also found at the body's various systems intersection, allowing communication and coordination between different cell types. For example, at the site of an injury, cannabinoids can be found performing three functions: 1) Decreasing the release of activators and sensitizers from the injured tissue, 2) Stabilizing the nerve cell to prevent excessive firing, and 3) Calming nearby immune cells to prevent the release of substances that promote inflammation. There are three different mechanisms of action on three different cell types for a single purpose: to minimize the pain and damage caused by the injury.

With its complex actions in our immune system, nervous system, and all of the body's organs, the endocannabinoid system is literally a bridge between body and mind. When we understand this system, we can begin to see a mechanism that explains how states of consciousness can promote health or disease.

Cannabinoid receptors are found all throughout our bodies, giving them a wide variety of functions. However, certain receptors are more concentrated in specific regions. CB1 receptors are most abundant in the brain, specifically in the central nervous system. CB2 receptors are more often found in immune cells, the gastrointestinal tract, and the peripheral nervous system.

The diversity of receptor locations shows just how important endocannabinoids are for day-to-day bodily functions. They help regulate the following:

- ✓ Sleep
- ✓ Appetite, digestion, hunger
- ✓ Mood
- ✓ Motor control
- ✓ Immune function
- ✓ Reproduction and fertility
- ✓ Pleasure and reward
- ✓ Pain
- ✓ Memory
- ✓ Temperature regulation

Endocannabinoids are the chemical messengers that tell your body to get these processes started and when to stop. They help maintain optimal balance in the body (homeostasis). When the ECS is disrupted, any one of these things can fall out of balance. When the ECS is imbalanced, it is thought to contribute to various conditions, including fibromyalgia and irritable bowel syndrome.

When the ECS is diseased, it is called *"Clinical Endocannabinoid Deficiency"*. The idea is this: when the body does not produce enough endocannabinoids or cannot regulate them properly, you are more susceptible to illnesses that affect one or more of the functions previously listed.

One unique factor separating cannabis from other illegal drugs is that the human body is equipped with an innate brain system that reacts to the THC and CBD enzymes. It is responsible for many body functions, including cognition, emotions, motor coordination and movements, appetite, and reaction to responses. And, unlike other illegal chemicals that create active damages to the neural receptors (for example, drugs like crystal meth and LSD burn a hole in the brain by damaging neurons and brain cells that can be shown in x-rays photos), the cannabinoids are natural and have no physical damage to the human brain and body. In fact, human breast milk naturally contains many of the same cannabinoids found in cannabis. These chemicals are actually extremely crucial for development, such as inducing nutrition intake, stimulating brain cell formation, and protecting body cells from harmful bacteria, viruses, and even cancer formation.

2. Public Knowledge Of Cannabis

Here is an important question to ponder: Why do we know more about man-made, synthetic drugs and pharmaceuticals than we do about cannabis, a natural plant, and its medicinal benefits? History shows quite a bit of documented evidence on the numerous medicinal benefits of cannabis. Did you know:

- Queen Victoria: She used cannabis as a pain relief for menstrual cramps. During the 1800s, Dr. William O'Shaughnessy was a pioneer of the medicinal use of cannabis in Europe. His influence on Sir J. Russel Reynolds prompted Reynolds' prescription of it to Queen Victoria. He is quoted as stating: *"When pure and administered carefully, cannabis is one of the most valuable medicines we possess."*
- George Washington: He grew hemp plants in abundance; it is said that Washington used it to alleviate his suffering with toothaches.
- John. F. Kennedy: He smoked cannabis to relieve his severe back pain.
- Chinese medicine has documented using cannabis to treat various pain problems like gout, rheumatoid pain, and a sedation for surgeries.

- Current Chinese pharmacies still sell a mild hemp drink during the summer to prevent heatstroke and stimulate the appetite.

These are just a few of countless examples of how cannabis has been used medicinally. Nevertheless, ever since cannabis was banned as an illegal drug in 1938, scientific research was halted in the United States until recent years due to the changing regulations towards medicinal usage. Still, the results of the research and studies are slanted towards the negative effects of cannabis.

Despite the negative propaganda surrounding cannabis use, the good news is that, with the increasing amount of treatment studies performed by hospitals and health science research laboratories all over the world (by countries where marijuana has been legalized), more and more discoveries of the benefits of this plant are coming to the forefront.

The U.S. government has classified cannabis as a "Schedule 1" Drug. The definition of a Schedule 1 drug is: *"Substances or chemicals that are defined as drugs with no currently accepted medical use and a high potential for abuse."* In the subsequent chapters of this book, we will see that this current classification is simply untrue as it relates to cannabis having "*no currently accepted medical use*."

Is Marijuana a Gateway Drug?

Many fear-based myths are surrounding the use of marijuana, one of those myths purports that marijuana is a "gateway drug". This phrase became popular in the 1980's; the assumption is that those who have used other drugs like heroin or cocaine started with marijuana – even though there is little to know evidence that marijuana is actually *causative* as it relates to other drugs. It is also worth noting that although there are no reported cases of fatal overdose with marijuana usage, there is such a thing as "overuse" and even mild symptoms of withdrawal due to excessive use. Another additional and very important aspect to mention regarding medicinal cannabis use is that it is virtually impossible to fatally overdose on it.

Marijuana and The Media/Movie Industry

The negative stigma and propaganda against cannabis use as purported by the movie industry began many decades ago to influence the masses against such usage. During the early 1900's several movies about marijuana were produced and portrayed the *assumed* tragic and/or dangerous eventualities. Many of us have heard of comedic movies such as Cheech and Chong's "Up in Smoke" and perhaps are familiar with other movies such as "Friday," "High On the Range," and "Reefer Madness."

Oftentimes Hollywood portrays the "typical" marijuana user as a rambling, bumbling unemployed idiot or hippy that binge watches T.V. in a psychedelic stupor, but with the growing trend of medicinal marijuana users, as well as responsible users, the landscape is slowly but surely changing. Let's take a brief look at some of the earlier movies created on this subject as well as some current statistics as they relate to media and marijuana use.

High On the Range (1929)

Several years before the making of "Reefer Madness", which created mass hysteria and a gross misunderstanding of marijuana to mainstream America, audiences were shown a silent short film called "High on the Range" created in 1929. The story features a man named Dave, a naive rancher who becomes a murderer after smoking less than a full joint.

Reefer Madness (1936)

This movie was intended to be a cautionary tale to make parents aware of the dangers of marijuana use, dangers such as addiction and insanity (madness). The story centers around a high school principal who shares a tale of two marijuana distributors who get several teenagers "hooked" on marijuana and are eventually met with several life-shattering tragedies, including reckless driving that leads to a car accident and an accidental shooting leaving a teenager dead.

Marijuana (1936)

"Reefer Madness" was not the only anti-marijuana movie made in 1936; one year before Federal Cannabis Prohibition became law in America, the film "Marijuana" purported itself as an exposé that divulged previously unheard of orgies and youths' debauchery. In short, producers pitched the movie on sex appeal and delivered such by having a group of party-goers skinny dip after smoking what they called "giggle weed". From there, it's all downhill for the main character – a young girl that smoked weed, got pregnant, and one of her friends drowns in the ocean; later, she turns from being an innocent girl to a calloused kingpin and heroin addict.

It is important to note that the impetus behind large corporations and the government's interference with the legalization of cannabis is money. William Randolph Hearst, who controlled a significant portion of news media in his day, vehemently supported the criminalization of marijuana primarily because his paper-producing companies were being replaced by hemp… FOLLOW THE MONEY!

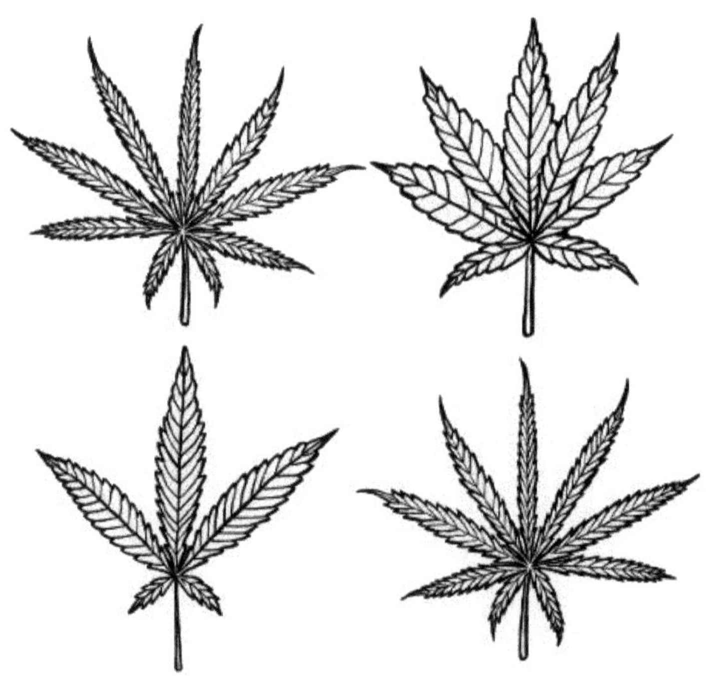

3. Types Of Cannabis

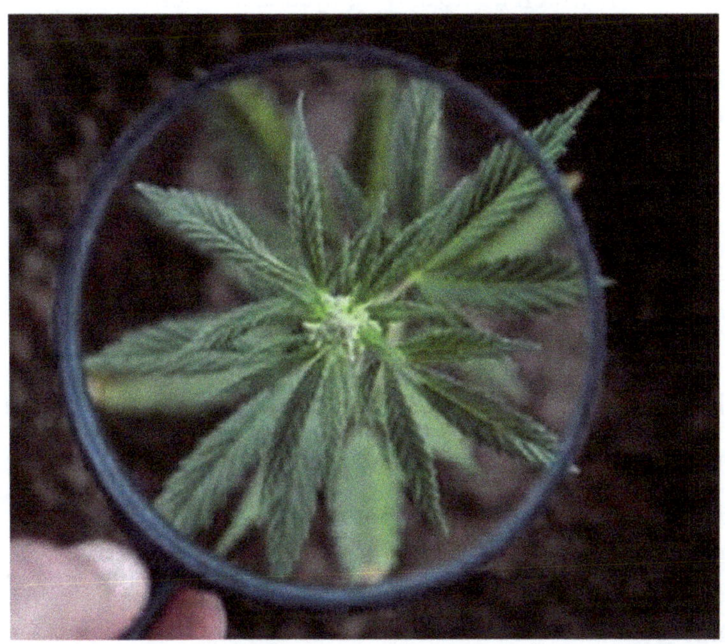

Sativa, Indica, and Hybrid

Perhaps you have heard the terms *Cannabis indica*, *Cannabis sativa*, or *Cannabis hybrid* in conversation or from various media outlets and informative articles. Even though all these species of cannabis are indeed marijuana, they differ slightly in a few ways; the first way is in their appearance.

The sativa plants tend to have longer, narrower leaves, whereas the indica plants tend to have wider, broader leaves. As for hybrids – they are a crossbreed between indica and sativa plants, the appearance can vary from strain to strain depending on the genetic makeup. Cannabis sativa is the plant from which hemp and marijuana are born.

As it relates to effect, the major qualities of sativa strains are as follows:

- Anti-depressant
- Anti-anxiety
- Increase of focus and creativity
- Treats chronic pain

The medicinal properties derived from sativa plants usually have a lower CBC count and a higher THC count. However, this can vary depending on the particular strain.

Some of the major qualities that indica plants possess are:

- Muscle relaxation
- Decrease of nausea
- Increase in appetite
- Increase in dopamine (a neurotransmitter that regulates the brain's pleasure centers)
- Increased mental relaxation

Besides their appearance, indica and sativa plants tend to have different effects on the user. These effects are indicated as follows:

Indica	Sativa
Relaxing, calming	Energizing, uplifting
Pain numbing	Thought inducing
Body buzz (similar to alcohol)	Hallucinogenic, Intellectually stimulating
Sleep inducing	Lightheadedness
Best for evening use	Best for daytime use

In appearance, indica plants are short, typically under six feet, and have fat deep green leaves. Indica mainly originates from Afghanistan, Pakistan, India, and the surrounding areas. The high from a quality indica strain leaves you relaxed and social. The stronger varieties will numb your body and put you to sleep. Great for relaxation, stress relief, or unwinding on your couch.

On the other hand, sativa plants can grow as high as twenty-five feet tall, but most plants stay under twelve feet. Its long, thin, light green leaves became the stereotypical marijuana symbol or icon. As noted in the table, the high from sativa strains are often described as uplifting and energetic. These are great for daytime use and a favorite for medicinal users because of its pain-relieving properties.

However, there are actually no scientific studies to confirm these body effect differences and accuracy between the two types of cannabis. These are solely based on the personal opinion of cannabis users in general. Moreover, history suggests a much simpler difference between indica and sativa. According to the original classification, Cannabis indica was named by the biologist Jean-Baptiste Lamarck. He noticed that the cannabis plants from India appeared to be different from the cannabis plants in Europe. To separate the two, he labeled Cannabis indica for the cannabis in India and sativa for the cannabis in Europe. Although the indica plants may have had a higher THC content at one point in time, the sativa plant may have had a higher CBD content. Due to the mixing of gene pools in the strain breeding process, many plants with varying amounts of CBD and THC chemicals have been produced. In the current cannabis gene pool, one may find certain sativa strains rich in THC and indica strains with low THC content.

Generally speaking, in today's cannabis products, indica strains are typically the ones that have a high THC to low CBD ratio, while sativa strains typically have a high CBD content to low THC content ratio, and hybrid strains usually have a 50:50 ratio of THC to CBD contents. Even within a specific strain of cannabis, you can still find variations of the cannabinoid contents because of the heredity combination as expressed in the female plants.

Since there is such a large number of cannabis strains, it can be difficult for consumers to find the right strain for their needs. In order to help prevent being overwhelmed by an abundance of choices, many of the products, such as dried flowers, tinctures, and edibles will indicate the amount of THC and CBD content; this way, consumers can pick out the product(s) that match their individual needs. Here is an example, an individual can choose a product that is higher in THC to get pain relief and to help with sleep apnea, but another individual may choose a product that is higher in CBD if they suffer from depression, while others may even opt for a hybrid strain to help with pain management but still want an "upbeat" sensation without the sleepy after effects.

4. Cannabis As Treatment For Various Illnesses

Cannabis use for medicinal purposes is becoming more and more widespread as more and more people (including children) with various illnesses have run into the proverbial "brick wall" as it relates to the ineffectiveness of synthetic drugs/pharmaceuticals, not to mention the negative side effects of various man-made drugs. How many of us have seen or heard commercials for prescription drugs that are promoted to help with a specific illness but are given a myriad of potential side effects at the end of the commercial? Who wants to take a drug that will *"heal"* you of one illness only to possibly receive several more illnesses as a result? Not to mention the fact that most pharmaceuticals don't truly heal the patient but rather only mask and/or suppress the symptoms?

Cancer

Some may wonder how popular medical cannabis is among cancer patients in states that have legalized both medical and recreational use. Researchers at the National Cancer Institute – a designated cancer center in the state of Washington, set out on a journey of discovery.

Researchers conducted a survey at the Seattle Cancer Care Alliance and published their findings in the medical journal on cancer; the article states that researchers found out that 74% of the eligible participants who completed the survey wanted information on medical marijuana from cancer care providers. However, their chances of receiving that information were very slim.

According to the same study, fewer than 15% of those patients received information about medical marijuana from their cancer physician or nurse. Most information was sought out from friends, family members, newspaper articles, other cancer patients, and cannabis resource websites such as Leafly. Only 73 out of the 926 patients who completed the survey (8%) said they did not want to receive any information on medical marijuana.

PTSD (Post Traumatic Stress Disorder)

Signs of distress are a commonplace reality for literally hundreds of thousands of veterans nationwide and also for hundreds of thousands of New Yorkers who suffer from PTSD. The physical and emotional stress of PTSD can be torture, but studies suggest medical marijuana can alleviate symptoms of anxiety, nausea, flashbacks, and insomnia.

The National Center for PTSD estimates that 8 percent of the U.S. population will suffer from PTSD at some point in their lives, and with nearly 20 million residents per state, as many as 1.6 million New Yorkers have experienced a severe, emotionally traumatizing event and are struggling to cope with PTSD. The potential for those numbers to increase becomes greater as we learn more about the causes, triggers and improve diagnoses.

Veterans and service members are most often associated with PTSD, but it is also common among firefighters and first responders, victims of domestic violence, violent crimes, sexual assault, and survivors of traumatic accidents and natural disasters such as tornadoes, earthquakes, floods, and the like.

Just this year, in February 2019, Dr. Sue Sisley and her team, with the California-based Multidisciplinary Association for Psychedelic Studies, completed a study of four different strengths of smoked cannabis on treatment-resistant PTSD. Over a period of nine months, Dr. Sisley's research team observed 76 veterans diagnosed with chronic, intractable PTSD.

Each veteran was randomly assigned to receive one of the four types of cannabis with varying levels of THC and CBD content as well as a placebo, fiber-variety "hemp" cannabis. Each participant was instructed to smoke two of the four types over a three-week period – up to 1.8 grams each day. Participants could use as much or as little as they needed, and between each session, will go through a two-week "clean" period where no cannabis use will be permitted. During the study, the research team observed changes in the severity of PTSD symptoms and relied on a friend or family member to report on the health and well-being of the participants.

The study allowed researchers to better understand the potential risks and benefits of cannabis use among veterans with PTSD and aided in cannabis-based decision-making among patients and their physicians.

Alzheimer's Disease (A.D)

A.D. is a neurodegenerative brain disease that affects thinking skills, memory, and eventually causes difficulty with even the simplest of tasks. Some of the symptoms associated with A.D. include agitation, weight loss, and pain; these challenges create a significant decline in the quality of life.

Since 2006, numerous medical studies have shown THC to be helpful in slowing down the plaque formations responsible for Alzheimer's disease. By blocking the neural enzyme that produces the plaque, cannabis can greatly decrease the progression of the disease. In more recent studies, researchers have even stated that cannabinoids can actually protect individuals from developing Alzheimer's disease because of their anti-inflammatory properties as well as neurogenesis properties.

There is currently an important ongoing investigation taking place in Toronto, Canada, at the Sunnybrook Health

Sciences Centre; they are studying a substance called *nabilone*, a synthetic compound with properties similar to THC. The study aims to investigate potential safety and effectiveness in treating Alzheimer's disease (A.D.). Beginning in 2015, the study recruited 40 participants for 14 weeks of testing. Half the participants were given nabilone treatment for six weeks then switched to placebo at the midpoint. The other half of the participants began with the placebo then were switched to the nabilone at the midpoint. Both groups took a one-week break from the medication or placebo at the midpoint. Researchers observed the effects of nabilone on agitation as well as other neuropsychiatric symptoms like cognition, pain, inflammation, and vital signs.

Although antipsychotics are well-studied and typically recommended, they are only modestly effective and have potentially severe side effects. Nabilone has shown beneficial results in other studies, and researchers speculate that it could be effective for symptoms of A.D. Although nabilone is a single molecule compound (compared to the many compounds in the cannabis flower), results from studies like this may give insight into how THC may benefit Alzheimer's patients.

Parkinson's Disease (P.D)

P.D. is a progressive and permanent condition that affects the nervous system. The Colorado Department of Public Health assigned the University of Colorado to study the tolerability and effects of cannabidiol (CBD) on tremors associated with Parkinson's disease (P.D.). Since marijuana became legal in Colorado, individuals with P.D. have self-medicated with marijuana, yet no studies show whether it's efficient in treating symptoms; however, animal studies using CBD suggest that it reduces anxiety, decreases psychotic symptoms, and improves both motor and non-motor symptoms in P.D.

This study will first determine a tolerable dose of CBD in 10 patients with P.D. and measure changes in vital signs or negative effects as doses increase from a baseline level to 20 mg of CBD. Subsequently, the effects of CBD on cognition, anxiety, sleep, fatigue, mood, pain, motor, and non-motor P.D. signs will be measured.

Most current therapies of P.D. are minimally effective and poorly tolerated. This detailed study is a step forward in examining the benefits and risks of CBD at specific dosages, providing much-needed information to physicians treating P.D. patients with cannabinoid medicine.

Osteoarthritis

Osteoarthritis is a painful, degenerative joint disease associated with the deterioration of cartilage. Currently, no drugs are available to control the progression of this disease, therefore the therapeutic approaches for osteoarthritis are limited other than typical analgesic treatments that have restricted efficacy. Increasing evidence from preclinical studies supports the interest of the endocannabinoid system as an emerging therapeutic target for osteoarthritis pain. Indeed, pharmacological studies have shown the antinociceptive effects of cannabinoids in different rodent models of osteoarthritis, and compelling evidence suggests active participation of the endocannabinoid system in the pathophysiology of this disease. The ubiquitous distribution of cannabinoid receptors, together with the physiological role of the endocannabinoid system in the regulation of pain, inflammation, and even joint function, further support the therapeutic interest of cannabinoids for osteoarthritis. However, despite the promising preclinical data, limited clinical evidence has been provided to support this therapeutic use of cannabinoids. This review summarizes the promising results that have been recently obtained in support of the therapeutic value of cannabinoids for osteoarthritis management.

Components Of Marijuana

THC (Tetrahydrocannabinol)

THC is mostly responsible for marijuana's psychological effects. Because cannabinoid receptors (the CB1 receptors and CB2 cannabinoid receptors) are mostly found in brain regions that are responsible for pleasure, coordination, time perception, memory, and thinking, these regions are activated when THC attaches to the receptors to create the euphoric feeling and impairment of coordination. THC has been shown to increase dopamine release and has powerful pain relief and sedation properties. It has also been shown to increase appetite and prevent nausea and vomiting, but at the same time, its interaction with CB1 receptors has been shown to increase metabolism and promote weight loss.

However, marijuana use can have other short-term side effects such as hallucination, tachyarrhythmia (cardiac arrest and/or heart failure), anxiety attack, and short-term memory impairment.

CBD (Cannabidiol)

This is the second most common cannabinoid found in many strains of cannabis, and there are certain strains of which the concentration of CBD is much higher than THC. In some rare strains, the ratio between the two cannabinoids is so significant that there are only traces of THC concentration, yet the CBD concentration is extremely high. Unlike THC, CBD has very little (if any) psychoactive effects, in other words, it does not cause a *high*, which has caused many "stoners" (a cannabis user that regularly gets high), and other consumers to ask: "*Well, what's the point?*" This question is typically asked by those that are not aware of all the benefits that CBD offers. The CBD chemical has shown to have antipsychotic properties that balance out the anxiety and panic attack effects THC can have on some individuals. It has also been demonstrated to improve wakefulness and work together with THC to suppress pain and spasm in muscles. When CBD alone is taken, it has been proven to be anti-epileptic, anti-inflammatory, and anti-anxiety. CBD can be used as a sedative and contains neuroprotective abilities to protect neurons and brain cells from various forms of damage. Furthermore, the U.S. government has stated that when CBD is used topically, it also has powerful anti-aging properties for skin cells.

In addition to CBD being an amazing anti-inflammatory (which makes it an ideal alternative to many over-the-counter pain medications), CBD comes in various forms such as oil, gels, gum, and supplements. CBD has also been known to bring relief from arthritis, backaches, and chemotherapy symptoms. It can help with nausea, migraines, depression, and anxiety.

It is important to note that in June 2018, the Food & Drug Administration (FDA) approved CBD oil as a therapy for epileptic seizures; this will be discussed further in a later chapter. Epidiolex is the first and only FDA-approved prescription of Cannabidiol.

CBN (Cannabinol)

This is the third most common cannabinoid and is actually a byproduct of the THC chemical breakdown. It has very few psychoactive and medicinal properties. CBN is typically found in poorly stored marijuana that has been kept in hot temperatures; despite this, CBN does indeed have other benefits; CBN causes sleepiness and is used as a sedative. It was also discovered to be effective as an anti-bacterial agent when applied topically.

THCA (Tetrahydrocannabinolic acid)

THCA, though it sounds very similar to THC, is very different in its components in that, like CBD, it is also non-psychoactive. While it is widely accepted that THC is the most prevalent chemical found in cannabis buds, it actually exists in the acidic form of THC acid (hence THCA). High heat is needed to convert THCA into the psychoactive THC form; this conversion process via heat is called *decarboxylation.* Even though THCA is not psychoactive, the benefit of this component is that it has been found to have the ability to regulate the immune system to desired levels (immunomodulation). Also, preliminary research of THCA has shown additional benefits such as treatment for nausea and loss of appetite and anti-inflammatory properties for conditions like arthritis. Further research of THCA is ongoing in order to substantiate these claims.

THCV (Tetrahydrocannabivarin)

Chemically speaking, THCV is very similar to THC; THCV is an appetite suppressant and anti-convulsive chemical. Even though it is psychoactive, it causes more of a "clear-head" euphoric effect, similar to CBD strains that have higher ratios.

Another interesting detail about CBD and THC is that they are both in hemp and marijuana and are the most famous components. As previously mentioned, cannabinoids aid in repairing and balancing our bodies through our endocannabinoid system. THC is the most famous property because it is the cannabinoid that causes the "high". CBD, THC, and all of the other cannabinoids are in the flowers, seeds, and stalks of the hemp and marijuana plants. One of the differences between Hemp and Marijuana is that hemp produces a higher CBD to THC ratio and marijuana a higher THC to CBD ratio, in other words, CBD is most prevalent in hemp, while THC is most prevalent in marijuana.

5. Central Nervous System – Tumors In Children

The University of Colorado is also conducting an additional observational study[1] in partnership with the Children's Hospital Colorado Center for Cancer and Blood Disorders. Over the course of a year, the team will observe 150 children between ages 2-18 that are diagnosed with Central Nervous System (CNS) tumors, who are self-medicating with cannabis while receiving treatment at CHCO.

During this study, the research team will administer questionnaires and use diaries to gather data on medical cannabis use, delivery methods, what strains are used, frequency and dosing amounts, and the financial impact on families. While controversial due to its involvement of minors and lax observation methods, this novel study will provide unprecedented statistical insight into how children with CNS tumors and their families use medical cannabis treatment. The results may provide helpful information that will influence the use of medical cannabis in other cancer patients.

---

[1] Foreman, N. K. (2017). Medical Marijuana in the Pediatric Central Nervous System Tumor Population - Full Text View - ClinicalTrials.gov. Clinical Trials. https://clinicaltrials.gov/ct2/show/NCT03052738?term=cannabis&recrs=af&draw=1

While there is evidence of the benefits of medical cannabis,[2] these new studies are helping researchers and physicians find exact dosages and application methods for specific ailments. The prohibition of research has been an obstacle for physicians, scientists, and patients alike. As opportunities for research open up, and as clinical data and continued anecdotal evidence accumulate, the knowledge gained from these studies will help patients struggling with serious medical conditions make informed decisions about using cannabis as medicine.

---

[2] Mechoulam, R, (2015). Cannabis - The Israeli perspective. *Journal of Basic and Clinical Physiology and Pharmacology,* 27(3). https://www.researchgate.net/profile/Raphael-Mechoulam/publication/282361085_Cannabis_-_The_Israeli_perspective/links/562c7b1c08aef25a2441d131/Cannabis-The-Israeli-perspective.pdf

6. Diabetes

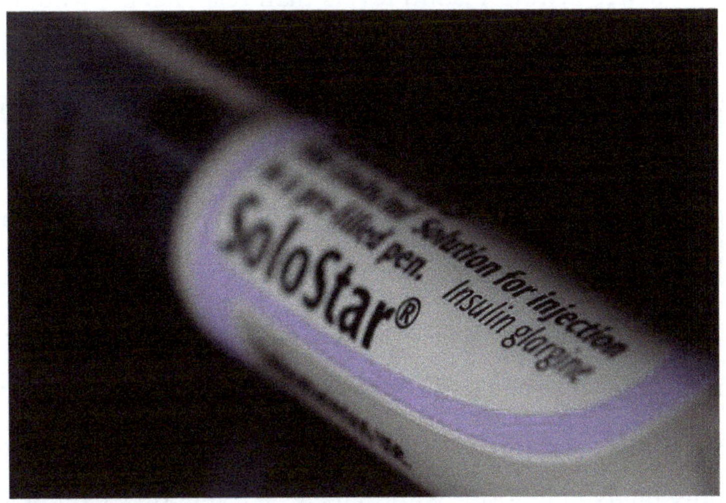

Preventative

Diabetes is associated with high levels of fasting insulin and insulin resistance and low levels of high-density lipoprotein cholesterol (HDL-C). In 2013, the results of a five-year study into the effects of cannabis on fasting insulin and insulin resistance[3] were published in the *American Journal of Medicine*. Of the 4,657 respondents, 2,554 had used cannabis in their lifetime (579 were current users, and 1,975 were past users), and 2,103 had never used the drug.

---

[3] Penner, E, A, Buettner, H, Mittleman, M. A, (2013). The Impact of Marijuana Use on Glucose, Insulin, and Insulin Resistance among US Adults. *CLINICAL RESEARCH STUDY*, 126(7). https://www.amjmed.com/article/S0002-9343%2813%2900200-3/fulltext

The researchers found that current users of cannabis had 16% lower fasting insulin levels than respondents who had never used cannabis and 17% lower levels of insulin resistance and higher levels of HDL-C. Respondents who had used cannabis in their lifetime but were not current users showed similar but less pronounced associations, indicating that the protective effect of cannabis fades with time.

Current cannabis users were found to have lower levels of insulin resistance than past users or non-users. The researchers also ran analyses on the data that excluded individuals diagnosed with diabetes. Even after excluding people with diabetes, current cannabis users were found to exhibit reduced fasting insulin and insulin resistance levels, indicating that cannabis can help prevent the occurrence of diabetes and control symptoms in diagnosed cases.

Lowers Insulin Resistance

Insulin resistance (I.R.) is a condition that causes cells to reject the normal mechanism of insulin[4], a hormone that is produced by the pancreas and is fundamental to the regulation of glucose metabolism. I.R. is associated with type 2 diabetes; in type 1 diabetes, the body is unable to produce insulin, while in type 2, insulin production is unaffected, but the cells are unable to process it. When cells become insulin-resistant, they are unable to absorb the

---

[4] "Insulin," n.d.

glucose needed to supply them with energy. The unused glucose builds up in the bloodstream–leading to hyperglycemia.

The authors of the 2013 study found that current users of cannabis had a mean I.R. of 1.8, compared to 2.2 for past users and 2.5 for those that had never used cannabis. Current cannabis users were also found to have lower levels of blood glucose compared to past users and non-users. Current users had mean blood glucose levels of 99.7 mg/dL, compared with 100.6 mg/dL for past users and 103.5 mg/dL for non-users. However, the precise mechanism via which cannabinoids exert their effects on I.R. has thus far not been determined.

Helps Prevent Obesity

Obesity, high body mass index (BMI), and large waist circumference are all linked to diabetes risk. Various studies have been conducted on the relationship between cannabis use and BMI, with conflicting results. A 2005 study[5] on young adults found that cannabis use was not associated with changes in BMI, whereas two large national surveys found

---

[5] Rodondi, N, Pletcher, M J, Liu, K, (2006). Marijuana Use, Diet, Body Mass Index, and Cardiovascular Risk Factors (from the CARDIA Study). *PREVENTIVE CARDIOLOGY*, 98(4). https://www.ajconline.org/article/S0002-9149%2806%2900817-4/fulltext#secd15695734e2045

lower BMI[6] and decreased levels of obesity[7] in cannabis users despite higher-than-average daily consumption of calories. The 2013 study found that current cannabis use was associated with smaller waist circumferences than in past or non-users.

While the mechanism underlying the complex relationship between the endocannabinoid system, obesity, and diabetes has not been fully established, a 2012 study[8] demonstrated that obese rats lost significant weight and experienced an increase in pancreas weight after exposure to organic cannabis extract. The increase in the weight of the pancreas indicates that the beta cells of the pancreas (which are responsible for the production of insulin) are protected by the presence of cannabinoids – in type 1 diabetes, an autoimmune response destroys the beta cells, so providing protection to them may help to control the disease.

---

[6] Smit, E, Crespo, C J, (2001). Dietary intake and nutritional status of US adult marijuana users: results from the Third National Health and Nutrition Examination Survey. *National Library of Medicine*, 4 (3). https://pubmed.ncbi.nlm.nih.gov/11415485/

[7] Strat, Y L, Le Foll, B, (2011). Obesity and cannabis use: results from 2 representative national surveys. *National Library of Medicine*, 174(8). https://pubmed.ncbi.nlm.nih.gov/21868374/

[8] Levendal, R-A, Schumann, D, Donath, M, Frost, C L, (2012). Cannabis exposure associated with weight reduction and β-cell protection in an obese rat model. *National Library of Medicine*, 19(7). https://pubmed.ncbi.nlm.nih.gov/22421529/

May Treat Diabetes-Induced Neuropathy

People with diabetes often experience nerve disorders as a result of their disease. Nerve damage often affects the peripheries such as the hands and feet but may occur in any organ or region of the body. The damage may be symptomless, but pain, tingling, and numbness accompany the disorder in many cases. As with many forms of nerve pain, diabetic neuropathy can be hard to treat with conventional analgesics; however, there is evidence to indicate that cannabis may have a role to play here too.

A study published in 2009[9] investigated the antinociceptive (pain-reducing) effects of cannabidiol extract in cases of diabetes-induced neuropathy in rats. The authors found that repeated administration of CBD extracts "significantly relieved" mechanical allodynia (a painful response to non-painful stimuli) and restored normal perception of pain without inducing hyperglycemia. The treatment was also found to protect the liver against oxidative stress (which is believed to be a major contributing factor to developing neuropathy) and increase levels of nerve growth factor to normal levels. Current cannabis users had

---

[9] Comelli, F, Bettoni, I, Colleoni, N, Giagnoni, G, Cost, B, (2009). Beneficial effects of a Cannabis sativa extract treatment on diabetes-induced neuropathy and oxidative stress. *National Library of Medicine,* 23(12). https://pubmed.ncbi.nlm.nih.gov/19441010/

lower blood glucose levels than past or non-users (© Bodytel)

However, studies on humans have thus far yielded less positive results. Also, in 2009, a randomized controlled trial investigated the ability of G.W. Pharmaceuticals' Sativex spray to ameliorate the symptoms of diabetes-induced peripheral neuropathy[10]. Thirty subjects were administered with either Sativex or placebo; pain scores improved significantly across the board, but the effect of Sativex was not found to be significantly greater than that of the placebo.

May Treat Diabetic Retinopathy

Up to 80% of diabetes patients who have had the disease for over a decade acquire a complication known as diabetic retinopathy (DRP). The cells of the retina are progressively damaged. This condition is responsible for approximately 12% of new cases of blindness each year in the USA.

DRP is associated with a glucose-induced breakdown of the blood-retinal barrier, a network of tightly packed cells that prevent unwanted substances in the blood from entering retinal tissue. This breakdown causes neural tissue to be

---

[10] Selvarajah, D, Gandhi, R, Emery, C J, (2010). Randomized Placebo-Controlled Double-Blind Clinical Trial of Cannabis-Based Medicinal Product (Sativex) in Painful Diabetic Neuropathy. *American Diabetes Association*, 33(1). https://care.diabetesjournals.org/content/33/1/128.short

exposed to neurotoxins and increases the chance of bleeding within the retina.

It is thought that the pro-inflammatory immune response and oxidative stress processes have a key role to play in the breakdown of retinal cells–and there is evidence that Cannabidiol, with its known ability to combat both oxidative stress and inflammation, may be useful in treating the disorder. In a 2006 study published in the *American Journal of Pathology*, diabetic rats were administered with CBD and tested to determine the rate of retinal cell death[11]. It was shown that treatment with CBD significantly reduced oxidative stress and neurotoxicity–including levels of tumor necrosis factor-a, a substance known to be involved in the inflammatory response–and protected against retinal cell death and the breakdown of the blood-retinal barrier.

---

[11] El-Remessy, A B, Al-Shabrawey, M, Khalifa, Y, (2006). Neuroprotective and Blood-Retinal Barrier-Preserving Effects of Cannabidiol in Experimental Diabetes. *The American Journal of Pathology,* 168(1). https://www.sciencedirect.com/science/article/pii/S000294401062086X

7. Can Cannabis Help Manage Diabetes?

Direct Benefits For Type 2 Diabetic Patients

Cannabis is very well known for the unstoppable "munchies" urge it induces. Most people would think that an increased caloric intake would result in a higher BMI. It would also be logical to assume that marijuana users tend to be overweight and prone to diabetes. Surprisingly, these two assumptions do not seem to apply to marijuana users. In order to determine whether or not the assumptions stand, an early medical correlation study was conducted to examine the effects of cannabis use on blood glucose level[12] and insulin level. In the study, 579 subjects out of 4657 total participants were marijuana users. These 579 participants showed a lower tendency to have diabetes than non-marijuana users. What is even more intriguing is that cannabis users exhibit 16% lower levels of fasting insulin and 17% lower insulin resistance than subjects who do not use cannabis. The marijuana users were also found to have lower waist circumference and higher high-density lipoprotein cholesterol levels (commonly named the "good cholesterol"). This discovery answers how exactly cannabis can benefit type 2 diabetic and pre-diabetic individuals.

---

[12] Almekinder RN, E. Can You Guess Your Blood Sugar? *The Diabetes Council.* https://www.thediabetescouncil.com/can-you-guess-your-blood-sugar/

For individuals who suffer from obesity and type 2 diabetes[13], endocannabinoid imbalance may be one of the reasons why certain people have a hard time losing weight. It has been found that the endocannabinoid system has a role in regulating energy homeostasis, especially in the intra-abdominal adipose tissue. When the endocannabinoid system is over-regulated, excessive visceral fat accumulation in the stomach area may lead to reduced adiponectin release from the tissue. Adiponectin is a protein that is responsible for regulating glucose levels and fatty acid breakdown. The decreasing amount of adiponectin in the body can lead to insulin insensitivity and increase the chance of developing type 2 diabetes. This chain reaction can turn into a vicious cycle of insulin resistance, further endocannabinoid system activation, greater appetite, food-seeking behavior[14], and additional body weight and fat gain.

Unlike THC that creates the munchies effect, CBD can help suppress appetite and help individuals re-balance the endocannabinoid system by increasing the fat breakdown, increasing mitochondria activities, promoting metabolism, and decreasing fat storage. In a way, CBD changes the

---

13 Almekinder RN, E. Type 2 Diabetes: An Overview. *The Diabetes Council.* https://www.thediabetescouncil.com/type-2-diabetes-an-overview/

14 Almekinder RN, E. Diabetes Recipes: Low Carb Baking for the Holidays. *The Diabetes Council.* https://www.thediabetescouncil.com/type-2-diabetes-an-overview/

white-colored fat storage cells to beige-colored fat cells for energy making. So, not only is the fat much easier to be burned off, but the beige-colored fat cells also improve glucose tolerance by decreasing insulin resistance in the muscle and liver cells. Although it may not completely treat diabetes, CBD can alleviate the condition so those diabetic individuals can suffer from less blood glucose fluctuation and manage their blood glucose level with less medication.

Another factor that CBD is a suitable treatment option for type 2 diabetes is that insulin resistance is a great contribution to the disease. The anti-inflammatory ability can improve the body's sugar metabolism, suppress the short inflammation reaction to sugar ingestion, and provide many other health benefits to prevent complications that result from type 2 diabetes.

Aside from CBD, THCV can also be a weight loss aide for type 2 diabetes individuals who are obese and need to lose weight to better control their blood glucose level and prevent complications from arising.

Direct Benefits For Type 1 Diabetic Patients

The researchers demonstrated the potential of (CBD) to reduce the occurrence and delay the onset of Type 1 diabetes[15]. It was found that CBD exhibits anti-autoimmune abilities. Even though some non-specific immunosuppression medications have shown to be successful in preventing diabetes, they are not an ideal alternative. Suppressing the immune system in a general fashion for an extended amount of time would present a dangerous treatment. Moreover, these drugs were indicated to be working only temporarily in the clinic until resistance was acquired. The marijuana and diabetes research is a lot more promising. In fact, clinical studies have shown that CBD can save insulin-forming cells from damage so that normal glucose metabolism can occur. At the moment, scientists have successfully used CBD to reverse the autoimmune disease in mice that suffer from an early stage of type 1 diabetes. They are in test trials to transfer this knowledge into treatments for human patients so that CBD can be a cure for type 1 diabetes.

Although cannabis cannot cure type 1 diabetes currently, the THC enzyme can suppress the autoimmune attacks so that less insulin is needed to lower the blood glucose levels. At the same time, CBD has been found to reduce the inflammation of pancreatic cells, and THCV has been shown to improve glucose tolerance and increase insulin sensitivity

---

[15] Almekinder RN, E. Type 1 Diabetes: An Overview. *The Diabetes Council.* https://www.thediabetescouncil.com/type-1-diabetes-an-overview/

for type 1 diabetic individuals so that there is a possibility that less insulin is needed for the management, and the fluctuation of the blood glucose level is thus more manageable. To confirm these findings, another research was conducted in 2012 where obese rats lost significant weight and experienced an increase in pancreas[16] weight after exposure to organic cannabis extract. The increase in the weight of the pancreas indicates that the insulin producing pancreatic cells (known as beta cells) are protected by the presence of cannabinoids in type 1 diabetes.

For many type 1 diabetes patients, stress and anxiety are common problems that aggravate blood glucose level fluctuation. CBD and THC can help make stress much more manageable while boosting the overall energy level.

Direct Benefits For Pre-Diabetic Patients

In general, many prediabetes patients have similar problems like type 2 diabetic individuals; they are very likely to suffer from obesity, poor eating habits[17] and lack of exercise. Diabetes is associated with high levels of fasting insulin and insulin resistance and a low level of high-density lipoprotein cholesterol. 5-year studies that include 4,657

---

[16] Montgomery, B. The Death of A Pancreas. *The Diabetes Council.* https://www.thediabetescouncil.com/the-death-of-a-pancreas/

[17] Bowers, J, 5 Diet Habits Ruining Your Diabetes Control. *The Diabetes Council.* https://www.thediabetescouncil.com/5-diet-habits-ruining-your-diabetes-control/

participants have found that regular cannabis users have 16% lower fasting insulin levels than individuals who have never used cannabis. Cannabis users also have 17% lower levels of insulin resistance and higher levels of high-density lipoprotein cholesterol. These at-risk individuals may benefit from the health benefits offered by cannabis products. Many research studies have found that the average regular cannabis users tend to have a lower body mass index (BMI) than non-cannabis users. They also have a smaller waist circumference than non-cannabis users. At the same time, they have a lesser chance of developing type 2 diabetes than those who do not use cannabis. This study suggests that cannabis cannot only help control diabetes but also prevent the onset of diabetes.

8. Benefits For Complication Problems From Diabetes

Insulin Resistance

Insulin resistance (IR) is a condition that makes body cells reject the normal functioning of insulin, a pancreatic hormone that is essential to the regulation of glucose metabolism. Type 1 diabetic individuals are unable to produce insulin. Unlike type 1 diabetes, insulin production is unaffected in type 2 diabetes individuals. However, their body cells are ineffective at processing insulin or are unable to process it. When cells become insulin-resistant, they are incapable of absorbing the glucose needed to supply the cells with energy.

This reaction causes unused glucose to build up in the bloodstream. If left untreated, this causes a downward spiral of chain reaction that consequently causes hyperglycemia. A study conducted in 2013 has found that cannabis users have a mean insulin resistance of 1.8, whereas non-users have a mean of 2.2 insulin resistance. Current cannabis users are also discovered to have lower blood glucose levels compared to past users and non-users. These current cannabis users have a mean blood glucose level of 99.7 mg/dL. On the other hand, past users have a mean blood glucose level of 100.6 mg/dL, and past users have a mean level of 103.5 mg/dL. These conclusions highly suggest that cannabis can help suppress insulin resistance and help type 2 diabetic individuals in managing their blood glucose levels. However, more research is needed to better understand how exactly does cannabis help with this problem and whether it is THC, CBD, or other cannabinoids that actively help in reducing insulin resistance.

Cardiovascular Complications

The American Alliance for Medical Cannabis (AAMC) has suggested that cannabis can suppress arterial inflammation and prevent diabetic individuals from developing cardiovascular diseases. Cannabinoids also have the ability to keep blood vessels dilate so that circulation can be improved in the process. This can be great prevention for individuals who are prone to swelling of the feet due to poor circulation. It can also help with spider veins, varicose veins, night cramps, restless leg syndrome, blood clots, ankle swelling, lipodermatosclerosis, and panniculitis.

Skin Complications

One of the most common problems that diabetic individuals face is skin sensitivity and irritation complications. The cannabinoid inflammation suppression properties can help with skin inflammation problems. For those who tend to suffer from foot sores, rashes, and other skin irritation problems, cannabis can alleviate the complications and speed up the healing process. Several scientific studies have found THC to be beneficial to skin cancer. Other studies have documented the anti-aging and intense moisturizing properties of the cannabinoid. The sedation and pain relief properties can also help alleviate the uncomfortable sensations from the skin irritation. Without constant scratching and rubbing on the irritated area, the skin can heal faster to lessen the chance of further complications.

Neuropathy

Neuropathy refers to nerve damages caused by certain diseases or disorders. It is found in 60 to 70 percent of all individuals with diabetes. To be more specific, there are four types of diabetes-related neuropathy:

- peripheral neuropathy (nerve damages that are located in the hands, arms, legs, and feet),
- autonomic neuropathy (nerve damage that affects the nerves that regulate blood pressure, blood glucose levels, and the heart functioning),
- focal neuropathy (nerve damage to the head, torso, and legs specifically), and
- proximal neuropathy (it is sometimes referred to as diabetic amyotrophy; it is usually concentrated on one side of the body in the hips, thighs, and buttocks regions).

Neuropathy is simply one of the worst complications for diabetic individuals. Although several treatment options are available, none of them are sufficient in preventing neuropathy, let alone reversing the complications. While opioids and anticonvulsants do work as short-term treatments, they plateau at a 50% efficacy in pain reduction and are associated with severe side effects and addiction problems.

Several studies have shown vaporized cannabis to reduce pain and slow the advancing nerve damage of all four types of neuropathy. In some types, there was more than a 30 percent improvement without any significant impact on daily functioning or cognitive abilities.

The anti-inflammation property does not just stop there. The CBD and THC chemicals can also prevent nerve over-sensitivity and inflammation problems. Some health researchers have also suggested that the cell growth acceleration ability can even reverse the neuropathy damages.

Diabetic Retinopathy

Just like neuropathy, diabetic retinopathy is another common complication that makes life much more difficult for diabetic individuals. It has been shown in several studies that cannabidiol can work as a multi-tasker to protect the eyes from growing excess of leaky blood vessels (the number 1 symptom of diabetic retinopathy) and prevent retinal cell death. There are even some researchers who suggest that CBD may even have the cell growth ability to reverse the damage done by diabetes.

High Blood Pressure

High blood pressure is often a complication of Type 2 diabetes. Although medical marijuana does lower blood pressure, it also briefly raises heart rate after consumption. As a result, cannabis is not recommended for those individuals who have pre-existing heart conditions. Medical studies show that prolonged marijuana users can develop a tolerance for this side-effect, and they do not suffer any negative effects from the brief episode of quickened heart rate.

9. Other Health Benefits

Treatment For Psychological Problems

CBD is an effective treatment for mental health disorders such as anxiety, psychosis, and depression. Recent health studies have shown that neurogenesis (neural cell growth) is a crucial neurological process that effectively helps to alleviate stress. Similar to exercising, CBD facilitates neuron production. Some of the most well-known strains effectively treating anxiety and stress-alleviation are Cannatonic, Frank Ocean, and Ghost Rider. At the same time, CBD offers an instant energy boost for stressed individuals. Many high-functioning, anxious individuals have found CBD-heavy strains to be a new alternative to coffee without the jitteriness. It can also help to alleviate serious social anxiety.

For depressed individuals, the uplifting mood-enhancing ability of CBD has known to offer a positive reinforcement so that they can feel better about themselves and their current situation.

Treatment For Epilepsy

Cannabis can be a treatment to prevent seizures in individuals who suffer from severe epilepsy. Cannabinoids have been shown to significantly decrease both the severity and frequency of the seizures. In recent years, there have been a number of individual cases where cannabis has been proven to be beneficial to children who suffer from severe epilepsy disorder called Dravet's Syndrome. In these cases, the affected children have become much more stabilized after starting a daily CBD concentrated tincture regimen. One of the most famous cases is a 5-year-old girl named Charlotte Figi, who suffers from Dravet syndrome. In this case, a specialized CBD-heavy strain of cannabis called Charlotte's Web has been bred for her treatment. After the documentary on the case has been broadcasted on television and news articles, more children who suffer from similar health problems have started similar cannabinoid therapies and have seen greater improvement in physical and mental development within a short amount of time.

Cancer And Wasting Syndrome

One of the biggest discoveries of cannabis is that it can be a great treatment for various cancers. The Pacific Medical Center of San Francisco has made an important discovery that CBD is a powerful treatment to stop cancer cell proliferation, metastasis, and growth of tumors. A study done by Sean McAllister of the research center has shown breast cancer show that the number of cancer cells diminished as more CBD was applied. Essentially, CBD may be a generally effective way to switch off the cancer-causing gene, providing patients with a non-toxic therapy to treat aggressive forms of cancer.

There is one exception to the theory that CBD suppresses appetite, but it is a blessing as well. Many people who have difficulty eating due to stress or anxiety can use CBD to get rid of that sick feeling in their chest or stomach, allowing them to eat again once their anxiety subsides. Science research has shown that cannabis can reduce vomiting and nausea for patients who are going through chemotherapy. It also helps to improve appetite and promote eating.

Post-Traumatic Stress Disorder (PTSD)

Post-traumatic stress disorder is an anxiety condition caused by psychologically disturbing events such as sexual assault, severe accidents, and military[18] combat. Individuals who suffer from PTSD can exhibit a combination of symptoms such as constant flashbacks of the traumatic event, active social isolation, anxiety attacks, insomnia, constant nightmares, depression, and emotional instability. For these problems, CBD can help PTSD individuals to feel less anxious about their situation and feel motivated to carry on their daily activities.

---

[18] Almekinder, E. Can You Join the Military if You Have Diabetes? *The Diabetes Council.* https://www.thediabetescouncil.com/can-you-join-the-military-if-you-have-diabetes/

The THC enzyme can facilitate a calming effect during the nighttime to allow PTSD individuals to have a better sleep[19] without nightmares. Depending on the individual's needs and symptoms, several strains of the product may be needed to provide sufficient treatment.

Weight Loss

Even though cannabis has been known to initiate that "munchies" mode, scientists have noticed that cannabis users tend to have an average healthy weight and are in relatively good physical shape. But as explained earlier, not all strains of cannabis have the "munchies" effect. Although it is true that THC can increase appetite, CBD is known to suppress appetite. Also, further research studies have found that cannabinoids increase metabolism and promote more fat burning. At the same time, CBD is a great encouragement for users to get off the couch and exercise.

Treatment For Patients Who Suffered From Stroke

Research studies done by the University of Nottingham have indicated that cannabis can help protect the brain and neural damage caused by a stroke. By administrating Cannabis extract within a short duration after the stroke, the

---

[19] Fachetti, L. Link Between Sleep & Diabetes: Everything You Need To Know. *The Diabetes Council.* https://www.thediabetescouncil.com/link-between-sleep-diabetes-everything-you-need-to-know/

affected area by the stroke has significantly reduced in size. These findings are consistent amongst rats, mice, and monkey test subjects. Further studies in 2012 have revealed that CBD can actively block the glutamate neurotoxin from killing brain cells during and after a stroke. As a matter of fact, CBD has shown to be even more effective than vitamin E and A in blocking the glutamate neural damage. Similarly, this unique property allows CBD to help individuals who have suffered from concussions and brain trauma. A Harvard Psychiatry department professor Lester Grinspoon has even advocated that NFL football players should be allowed to take marijuana to prevent brain damage from the constant concussion and even avoid the development of Parkinson's and Alzheimer's diseases.

Glaucoma

Since the early 1970's, health research studies have found that cannabis lowers the intraocular pressure (IOP) in both normal people and patients who suffer from glaucoma. By decreasing the pressure, the cannabinoids allow less damage to the optic nerve that eventually causes vision loss. At the same time, it helps to alleviate various symptoms that are associated with glaucomas, such as eye pain and nausea.

Pain-Related Issues

Cannabis has a long history of being used as pain relief from chronic pain to muscle spasms to menstrual cramps.

As a matter of fact, a company backed by actor Whoopi Goldberg is in the works of creating a tampon that is infused with cannabinoids to alleviate menstrual cramps. There are also wide markets of cannabinoid-infused balms and lotions available as a topical pain relief aide. Individuals who are suffering from multiple sclerosis and other autoimmune debilitating conditions (e.g., lupus) can also benefit from the pain relief and anti-inflammatory properties of THC.

Inflammatory Bowel Diseases

Cannabis has also been proven to help patients who are suffering from inflammatory bowel diseases such as Crohn's disease, collagenous colitis, ulcerative colitis, and lymphocytic colitis. As these diseases stem from inflammation of the inner lining of the digestive tracts, the anti-inflammatory ability of the cannabinoid can drastically suppress the inflammation and pain relief for the intense pain associated with the damage. And in the process, the chemicals stop the digestive tracts from being over-stimulated and create more damages from the immune system attacking the inflamed areas.

Skin-Related Issues

In these few recent years, more and more cannabis-infused beauty products have come on the market as anti-aging skin products. These balms and lotions can actually treat skin irritation problems such as hives and rashes, acne (it moisturizes the skin while killing off germs and reducing inflammation), and eczema (it suppresses the redness and reduces irritation). As a matter of fact, cannabinoid cream can be used as an after-shave balm to slow down hair growth while calming the freshly-shaven skin from irritation.

Autism

Similar to treating severely epileptic children with CBD oil, children who suffer from severe cases of autism can show great improvement with CBD oil treatment. There have been numerous cases where a non-verbal child develops significant verbal skills and exhibits much more social interaction as little as three weeks.

Australian penny stock Zelda Therapeutics (ASX:ZLD) announced last week that it has completed an observation trial in Chile and is reporting successful results for treating core symptoms of autism with medical cannabis extracts. Zelda officials say they now plan to build on those results with clinical trials in the second half of 2017.

The trial, in collaboration with Chilean medical cannabis and alternative healthcare non-profit called Fundación Daya, aimed to treat core autism symptoms, including difficulties with social interaction, language, and repetitive behavior. The results found that in a cohort of 21 patients (median age of nine years and ten months), cannabis extracts were significantly more effective than the conventional medicines the children were using, including atypical antipsychotics.

Patients in the study were treated over 12 weeks and were examined by EEG, neuropsychological analysis, metabolism, and genetic tests. Those treated with cannabis extracts demonstrated significant improvements in at least one core symptom (social interaction, language, or repetitive behaviors) in 71.4% of cases and 66.7% of treated patients showing significant general overall improvement.

Harry Karelis, Executive Chairman of Zelda, was excited with the results, as he sees a promising future with treating autism symptoms with cannabis.

The results from this observational study are very exciting and support the anecdotal evidence we have, showing the positive effect medicinal cannabis has on treating autism symptoms," Karelis said in a statement.

"Zelda will use this baseline data to design its clinical trials and generate rigorous scientific data that validates the clinical benefit of medicinal cannabis," Karelis added. "We hope that in the near future, Zelda Therapeutics can provide an alternative treatment for sufferers of this condition which is of major global significance."

There is little scientific literature covering the use of cannabis to treat autism. In 2011, a study published in

Current Neuropharmacology demonstrated that Δ9-THC improved mobility and mood[20] in a breed of mice that exhibit autism-like behavior. However, a study in mice is a long way from solid peer-reviewed studies in humans.

Clinical trials are critical for establishing the safety and effectiveness of treatment but also for ensuring its acceptance by regulators like Australia's Therapeutic Goods Administration. In the case of cannabis as an autism treatment, the lack of published studies makes successful clinical trials all the more important for Zelda.

Treatment For Anxiety (CBD)

While we don't normally think of anxiety as desirable, it's actually a critical adaptive response that can help us cope with threats to our (or a loved one's) safety and welfare. These responses help us recognize and avert potential threats; they can also help motivate us to take action to better our situation (work harder, pay bills, improve relationships, etc.). However, when we don't manage these natural responses effectively, they can become maladaptive and impact our work and relationships. This can lead to

---

[20] S. Onaivi, E., Benno, R., Halpern, T., Mehanovic, M., (2011). Consequences of Cannabinoid and Monoaminergic System Disruption in a Mouse Model of Autism Spectrum Disorders. *Current Neuropharmacology,* 9(1). https://doi.org/10.2174/157015911795017047

clinically diagnosable anxiety-related disorders. We've all heard the saying, "stress kills". It's true!

Anxiety-related disorders affect a huge segment of our population—40 million adults (18%) in the United States[21] age 18 and older. In response, Big Pharma has developed numerous drugs to treat anxiety-related disorders, from selective serotonin reuptake inhibitors (SSRIs) like Prozac and Zoloft to tranquilizers (the most popular class being benzodiazepines such as Valium and Xanax).

Prostate Cancer

While the studies are ongoing in the medical research community as to just how effective cannabis-derived oils are in treating cancer, there is enough evidence to suggest it's worth considering as part of an overall treatment.

The non-recreational cannabis-derived oil is shown to minimize pain, benefit sleep and relieve stress and anxiety, all symptoms that come with cancer.

Dr. Zeid Mohamedali, a urologist in Port Alberni, spoke about cannabis and prostate cancer at the Prostate Cancer Support Group meeting. Mohamedali is a proponent that

---

[21] Anonymous. Any Anxiety Disorder. *National Institute of Mental Health.* https://www.nimh.nih.gov/health/statistics/any-anxiety-disorder

medical cannabis can benefit patients as part of their overall cancer treatment.

Leanne Kopp, executive director of the Island Prostate Centre, said: *"Cannabis is a big part of [Mohamedali's] medical practice, [particularly] its use of symptomatic care, our role is to continue education and to support all types of treatments."*

Cannabis And Covid-19

Since coronavirus outbreaks first began to make the news, cannabis consumers have been wondering whether cannabis will hurt or help with Covid-19. At the onset, few had answers, but more and more research has been pouring in to date. Strangely enough, the research points in both directions – it suggests that cannabis may have the potential to both help and harm in cases of coronavirus infection.

Most of the new evidence points to CBD or terpenes from cannabis as a treatment for "*cytokine storms*" – the dangerous over-elevation of cytokines and inflammation which has led to the deaths of many Covid-19 patients, but some research also suggests that general cannabis use might increase the risk for Covid-19 patients.

Experts say that both lines of research could be pointing to the truth – with cannabis impacting patients differently depending on how it's used and how severely they are infected with Covid-19.

COVID-19 has caused millions of deaths, closed international borders, and has some economies on the brink of collapse. This contagious respiratory disease can leave one with a fever, feeling fatigued, and struggling to breathe.

Researchers suggest that cannabis might help those with Covid-19 points to cannabis-derived chemical CBD as a potential treatment during severe cases of Covid-19.

Scientists from the University of Nebraska and the Texas Biomedical Research Institute first flagged the possibility in a peer-reviewed article[22] in Brain, Behavior, and Immunity. They noted out that CBD may help fight cytokine storms.

Cytokines are proteins in the body that play an important role in our immune response – increasing inflammation in reaction to infections. This is crucial in fighting off infections, but sometimes in severe infections, the body goes too far and releases too many cytokines into the blood too quickly – hence the term "*cytokine storm*", which causes high fever, too much inflammation (redness and swelling),

---

[22] Immun, B. B, (2020). SARS-CoV2 induced respiratory distress: Can cannabinoids be added to anti-viral therapies to reduce lung inflammation? *Elsevier Public Health Emergency Collection. 10.1016/j.bbi.2020.04.079*

severe fatigue, nausea, difficulty breathing, and in some cases death due to organ failure.

Researchers are particularly interested in CBD because it has the ability to reduce these inflammation-causing cytokines and thus potentially end the cytokine storms.

A new Canadian study provided some data highlighting that some cannabis strains could help reduce this type of inflammatory distress. The study showed that cannabis has the potential to curb the severity of some Covid-19 symptoms.

The study was done by researchers at Pathway Research Inc, the University of Calgary, and the University of Lethbridge; the participating scientists used artificial human models, exposing them to UV rays that cause induced inflammation.

Afterward, the human models were treated with seven different cannabis strains to note the efficacy in reducing inflammation. Three strains were deemed the most effective.

According to the study, these three strains significantly helped to reduce these inflammatory cytokine storms. It showed that cannabis could dramatically improve the condition of COVID-19 patients by reducing the cytokine storm and protect lung tissue from damage caused by inflammation.

10. Importance Of Cbd-Rich Strains

Unfortunately, most commercially available indica strains have been selected and bred for their high THC levels and psychedelic effects for the past 20 to 30 years. This has resulted in CBD being nearly bred out of the plant – most strains contain less than 1% CBD. And since CBD typically shows up under 1% in most strains, it is sometimes hard to find a plant with equally low THC percentages to avoid the 'high' patients experience from THC.

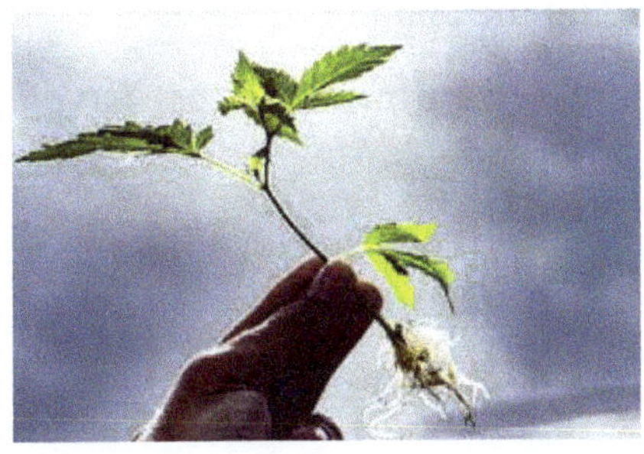

However, that does not mean that these CBD-rich strains don't exist! With so many medical discoveries on CBD, growers have realized that there are individuals who would benefit from a high CBD strain with very little THC content. As a result, many growers are now concentrating on CBD-rich strains for their medicinal benefits instead of pursuing gummy THC-covered strains. Consequently, CBD-rich strains are making a comeback.

As mentioned earlier, the Charlotte Web strain is a super CBD-rich strain that has only 0.3% THC content. Another popular CBD-rich strain is called ACDC, which has only 0.42% of THC content. This strain is popular for patients who suffer from PTSD, epilepsy, cancer, multiple sclerosis, and autism. Although growers are striving to come up with even better CBD-rich strains, there have been suggestions that a completely no THC strain cannot exist because it plays a role in the plant structure. The evidence can be seen in CBD-rich strains as the plants exhibit very weak stems and require much support to hold up the plant until harvest. This stem weakness is much more severe in plants that have a lower THC content.

11. Ways Of Consuming Cannabis

After hearing that there are so many advantages to cannabis, you may start to wonder if you need to smoke the herb in order to receive the benefits. The answer is no. There are numerous ways in which individuals can be medicated without hitting a lighter. Here is a list of ways cannabis can be consumed:

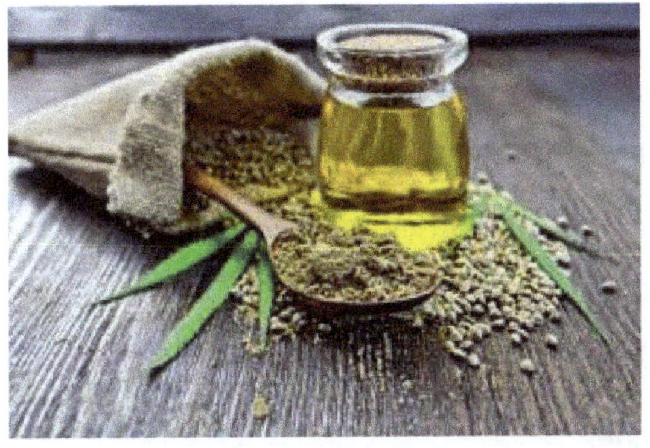

Smoking

This is the most original and simple method of consuming cannabis. The most common way is to grind up the dried female flower buds into fine granules, burn the content, and inhale the vaporized smoke containing the cannabinoids through a bong, pipe, paper-wrapped joint, and tobacco-leaf wrapped or cigar wrapping blunts.

For some individuals who want to intake less smoke, they may prefer smoking the Kief. Kief is a refined powder containing the trichrome of the flower buds and some leaves and flower residues. And when the residues are all sifted out, this super-refined trichrome powder is called hash or hashish.

Dabbing

The hash can be smoked with a bong or "dabbed" using a high heat device called a rig. Usually, the hash is further processed into a sticky oil substance, called wax (it can also be called shatter, budder, honey oil, and butane hash oil depending on the appearance of the concentrate and the method being used to process the hash) to be burned on the heating device or a vaping pen. This wax is super high in THC and CBD content and should not be used by beginners as the dosage is very high compared to smoking or vaping.

Vaporizer

This method is commonly known as vaping. Like nicotine vaporizers, the cannabinoids are extracted from the dried flowers into a concentrated oil (often called hash oil) through various methods. The heating coil then heats this oil in the vaporizer pen or machine to about 329 to 374F degrees, and the oil is turned into vapor for inhalation.

Tincture

Cannabinoids can be extracted from the flower buds by using alcohol or food-grade glycerin to create a concentrated, thick liquid solution. The most famous tincture is Rick Simpson Oil, originally produced from only indica strains of cannabis to treat cancer and tumors. In the last few years, rich CBD strains have also been processed into tinctures so that children can benefit from the cannabinoids without needing to inhale vapor or eat an edible. This method also allows a precise measurement of dosage for the treatment without any need for estimation.

Infusions

This category is quite similar to tincture. The only difference is that instead of using alcohol and food-grade glycerin to extract the cannabinoids, a fatty solvent is used for the extraction process. The solvent can be butter, cocoa butter, coconut oil, various cooking oil such as olive oil, milk, cream, and even non-edible skin moisturizing oils.

Edibles

The food-grade oil or cream infusions can then be eaten directly or made into an edible for consumption. Those food items that include these oil infusions or tincture infusions are all categorized as edibles. These days, you can find anything, like a wide range of edibles that are similar to desserts[23] and candy. Other edibles can include ice cream,

---

[23] Bowers, J. 9 Low Sugar/Carbohydrate Dessert Recipes (Diabetes Friendly). *The Diabetes Council.* https://www.thediabetescouncil.com/9-low-sugarcarbohydrate-dessert-recipes-diabetes-friendly/

pasta sauce, coffee creamer, syrup, and even chewing gum. For individuals who cannot ingest fat, dairy products, or alcohol due to various allergies or medical conditions, companies have produced capsules containing the extract for consumption.

Patch

Similar to a nicotine patch, various manufacturer companies have produced a cannabinoid patch for individuals who just wish to enjoy the benefits without even consuming any cannabis products. The cannabinoid-infused tampons are another variation from the same methods. Another variation works by an oral dissolve strip similar to a breath freshener strip.

12. Side Effects Of Marijuana

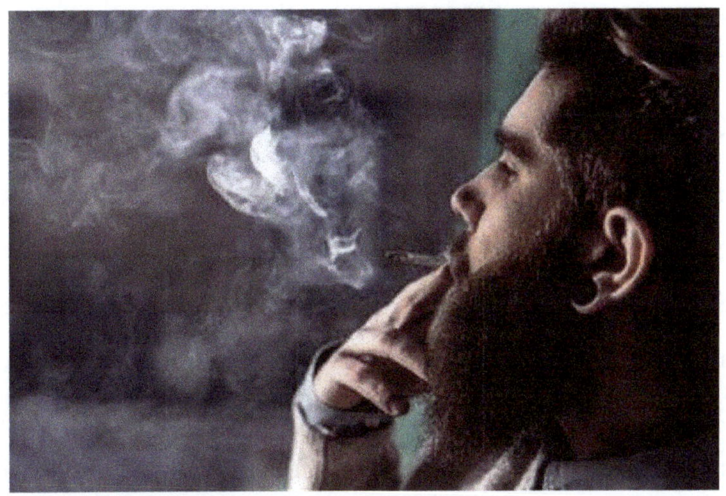

Because cannabis is still illegal under federal law in the United States and many parts of the world, there is still a limited amount of extensive research on the long-term effects of cannabis. According to the Drug Enforcement Agency in the United States, here are some of the possible short-term negative effects:

- coordination impairment
- lethargy and lack of energy
- drowsiness and sleepiness[24]
- disorientation
- faulty short-term memory

[24] Fachetti, L. Link Between Sleep & Diabetes: Everything You Need To Know. *The Diabetes Journal.* https://www.thediabetescouncil.com/link-between-sleep-diabetes-everything-you-need-to-know/

- lung damage if inhaled

Other common symptoms of consuming cannabis are dizziness, nausea, tiredness, and hallucinations.

It is also important to note that cannabis is not for everyone. Like any other medication treatment, each individual shows slightly different reactions from other people, based on their allergies and physical condition. Some people may exhibit allergy symptoms similar to pollen allergies (since cannabinoids are extracted from flower buds). In serious allergy cases, the individual may show swelling, excessive coughing, fever, and difficulty in breathing due to swelling of the air passages. Individuals who are allergic or sensitive to smoke vapor should avoid smoking cannabis. Because inhaling smoke can irritate the respiratory system, it should also be avoided by individuals who suffer from breathing-related conditions such as bronchitis and chronic obstructive pulmonary disease (COPD). And, as cannabinoids can produce a temporary increase in heart rate, individuals who suffer from high blood pressure or heart disease may want to avoid using cannabis unless they have consulted their doctors and have been advised otherwise. Those who have suffered from a stroke or heart attack must discuss the options with their doctors before trying any cannabis products. Individuals who suffer from a peripheral vascular disease caused by atherosclerosis should also avoid cannabis because elevated blood pressure may increase the chance of heart attacks, angina, and strokes. Moreover, because cannabis can cause dilation to the blood vessels, even the doctors do not know how it will react with your medications. Those individuals who are currently taking medications for their heart problems should also consult with their doctors[25] to discuss whether cannabis will interfere with their current medication.

Those suffering from hepatitis C and other conditions related to liver damage should also refrain from consuming cannabinoids in high doses daily because it causes further liver complications.

Individuals who are suffering from various mental health conditions should also avoid using cannabis. Although there is no direct correlation between mental illness and cannabis use, some research studies indicate marijuana may exacerbate symptoms associated with psychosis or schizophrenia. For those who wish to alleviate their mental illness conditions such as depression and bipolar disorder, these individuals should consult with their doctors[26] about their options.

---

[25] Montogomery, B. What You Want Your Doctor to Know About Your Diabetes. *The Diabetes Journal.* https://www.thediabetescouncil.com/what-you-want-your-doctor-to-know-about-your-diabetes/

[26] TheDiabetesCouncil Team, 7 Mistakes Doctors Are Making with Diabetes. *The Diabetes Council.*

Another important thing is that cannabis is not for children or teenagers unless absolutely necessary (for example, epilepsy and autism). While studies have shown that it does not pose as much damage as alcohol and many other illegal substances, questions remain about its possible influence on the developing brain. We know that the brain is under development until early adulthood (around 25 years old). During this volatile stage, the increased cannabinoids can potentially interfere with the growth and development of the endocannabinoid system and neural pathways. As a safety precaution, individuals should refrain from consuming cannabis until they reach the age of 25, unless they have a medical condition that can benefit from the cannabinoids.

Similarly, pregnant[27] women should avoid consuming marijuana, as they would for tobacco or alcohol. Any cannabis use must be stopped before and during pregnancy, as it can result in negative outcomes for both the mother and the baby. Although maternal use of cannabis during pregnancy[28] does not appear to be associated with low birth weight or early delivery, it may still affect the baby's neural

---

https://www.thediabetescouncil.com/7-mistakes-doctors-are-making-with-diabetes/

[27] Almekinder, E. Pre-existing Diabetes And Pregnancy. *The Diabetes Council.* https://www.thediabetescouncil.com/pre-existing-diabetes-and-pregnancy/

[28] Tomaselli, J. FAQs About Gestational Diabetes. *The Diabetes Council.* https://www.thediabetescouncil.com/gestational-diabetes-faq/

development related to the endocannabinoid system. It has even been suggested that babies who were exposed to cannabinoids during the fetus phase have shown an attraction towards cannabis in teenage and early adulthood. They are also shown to exhibit higher tolerance towards the herb. Unless there is an urgent medical need, the pregnant woman should not consume any Cannabis unless being advised by their physicians.

Long-Term Side Effects Of Cannabis

The long-term side effects of cannabis are still unclear in our current research on cannabis consumption. The main concern, for now, revolves around cognitive and memory problems. There have also been concerns for children, teenagers, and young adults exposing themselves to cannabis, as this may increase their chances of developing schizophrenia and various mental disorders such as anxiety disorder, bipolar disorder, and depression.

Even though the addictive properties of marijuana are relatively minimal compared to alcohol and other drugs, individuals who are prone to addictive behaviors may want to avoid cannabis because they may be more inclined to become dependent on the behavior.

Other long-term side effects may depend on the way cannabis is consumed. One evident long-term side effect is that smoking marijuana can cause rapid aging of the skin.

The THC smoke actually blocks the development of collagen from forming and causes your skin to age more quickly. This problem can be avoided by using vaporizers, consuming edibles, and other methods that do not include contact with the THC smoke. Similarly, smoking cannabis is similar to smoking tobacco use; the smoke damages the lungs and increases the chance of lung complications and cancer.

Effects Of Chronic Use Of Marijuana

The term chronic use can be confusing as there is no straight definition. According to scientific studies, chronic cannabis smoking is defined by an average of 9 joints per day for a duration of at least two years. Those who self-report as chronic cannabis smokers are found to be associated with excessive abdominal fat and insulin resistance in the adipose tissues. However, they do not suffer from fatty liver (also known as hepatic steatosis), insulin insensitivity, glucose intolerance, or reduced pancreatic beta-cell function. These findings are consistent with animal testing subjects. At the same time, clinical trials have found that heavy use of cannabis can actually reduce body weight, diminish low high-density lipoprotein levels, and decrease insulin resistance in human subjects.

Another important finding is that patients who suffer from chronic hepatitis C and use cannabis on a daily basis are highly associated with hepatic steatosis. There is actually evidence indicating that these patients may suffer from liver damage from chronic smoking of cannabis. This discovery suggests that individuals who suffer from diseases associated with liver problems should avoid cannabis use unless necessary.

There has been evidence that chronic cannabis users exhibit an elevated level of testosterone. This can lead to the development of acne and unusual hair loss.

13. Tolerance And Withdrawal

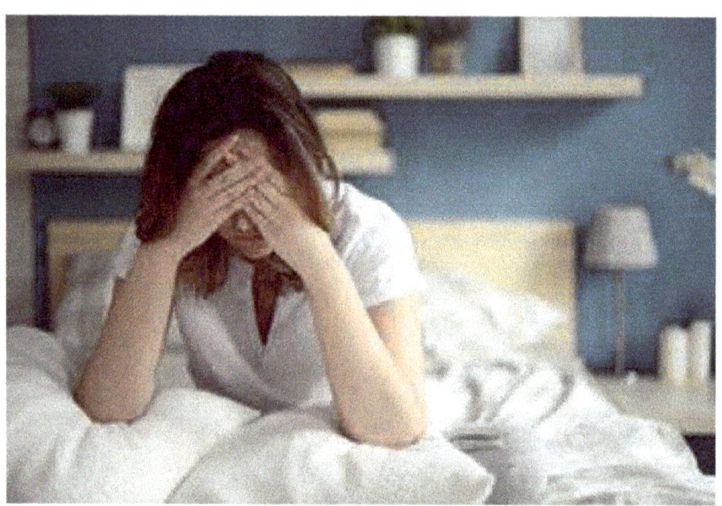

According to the United States Department of Health and Human Services, 129,000 emergency room visits were associated with cannabis use in 2011. This data does not mean that marijuana must be the direct cause of the visit. It can mean that the individual has consumed marijuana before the emergency room visit. What is more important is that there has never been a case of marijuana overdose in history. As a matter of fact, medical studies have shown that cannabis has a therapeutic index of 40,000:1. This index means that a person would need to take 40,000 times the normal dosage in order to be overdosed (morphine has a therapeutic index of 70:1).

Cannabis usually causes no tolerance or withdrawal symptoms, except in chronic daily users. Unlike alcohol, tobacco, various illegal drugs, cannabis withdrawal symptoms are much tamer and likened to those of an individual trying to quit coffee. In a survey of heavy users,

42.4% experiences withdrawal symptoms when they try to quit, such as craving, irritability, lack of energy, boredom, and anxiety. Those at the highest probability of developing cannabis dependences are those with a history of poor academic accomplishment, unusual behavior in childhood and adolescence, poor parental relationships, rebelliousness, or a parental history of alcohol and/or substance abuse problems.

How Much Is Too Much?

The effects of consuming cannabis vary from person to person, depending on the person's experience with cannabis, the type and amount consumed, the quality of the product, as well as the method of consumption frequently used. Those who enjoy using marijuana typically find it to be relaxing or mildly euphoric. Some find it makes them more social or outgoing, while other people claim that cannabis makes them feel jittery, uncomfortable, tired, or remote.

New Users Mistake

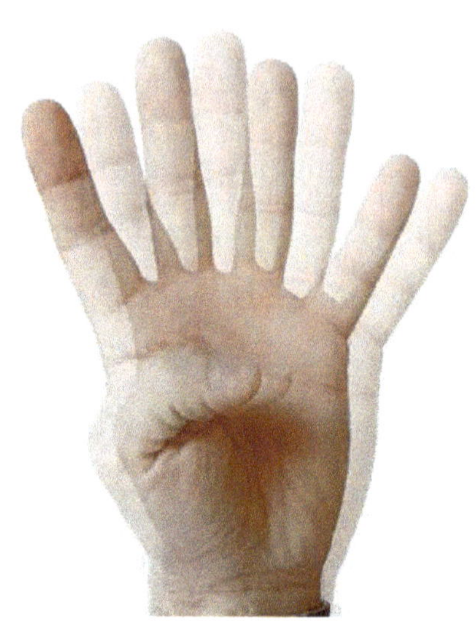

New users often experience different effects than more experienced users. The number one mistake for new users is to consume too much in one instance. This often leads to unpleasant feelings such as an increased heart rate, a sense of paranoia, cold sweat from the sudden adjustment of the sensory impairment, and stinging of the throat (especially individuals who have never smoked at all). Usually, a sense of panic induces a "bad trip", which includes similar symptoms of motion sickness and panic attacks due to over-breathing.

Not All Marijuana Products Are The Same

As explained in earlier sections, there are many different strains of cannabis. Even within the same strain of cannabis, the potency of the flower buds can differ based on the seed quality, the seed's DNA makeup (seeds coming from the same mother plant can express different phenotype expressions), and the growing process.

Dried Flower Buds:

Each strain of marijuana is different, varying in physical appearance and color, smell, and taste (names are often associated with their special features; for example, the Skunk strains smell like Skunk, the Purple Urkle is named for its purplish hue color buds, and Pineapple Express smells like pineapples). Inexperienced users should begin by consuming ONLY a small amount, such as one or two small puffs. Smoking and vaporizing have an immediate effect that can intensify quickly (usually within 10-15 minutes). Instead of taking more puffs, wait at least 20-30 minutes before using more. This way, you can gauge how one puff is affecting you. If you are vaping, keep in mind that the dosage is more potent in one puff. So, go even slower.

Concentrates:

These are highly concentrated forms of cannabis, such as hashes, Kief, oils, and waxes, which are created by extracting cannabinoids from the flowers and leaves of cannabis plants. If you are comparing marijuana to alcohol, flowers are analogous to a light beer and concentrate to hard liquor. If you are a beginner, never attempt to consume concentrates without being supervised. Even experienced users can easily misjudge the dosage and find themselves stuck to the couch. If you are trying concentrates for the first time, begin with a VERY small amount and wait at least 30 minutes before taking another dose.

Inhaling Vs. Ingesting Marijuana

It is essential to recognize that there are two important differences between consuming cannabis via inhaling and ingesting:

- Ingesting cannabis products usually produces much stronger and longer-lasting effects. The effects can take up to thirty minutes to two hours to start after consumption, and the "high" can last for a couple of hours.
- Inhaling marijuana is immediate, and the effects peak within ten to fifteen minutes. Compared to ingesting, the effect of inhaling cannabis can wear off within as early as one hour.

Things To Consider For Individuals Who Use Medical Marijuana To Treat Diabetes And Other Health Issues

Apart from the basic considerations already mentioned, there are some things to consider regarding your diabetes conditions. Here are some additional tips to keep in mind:

- **Be Aware Of Changed Perception** – Just like alcohol, you feel slightly unbalanced and experience blurry vision when you are under the influence of a mind-altering substance. During this time, you may not be able to recognize if you are feeling hypoglycemia and hyperglycemia. The increased heart rate may also confuse your judgment about feeling "high" or experiencing an episode of hypoglycemia.

- **Check Your Blood Glucose Level Frequently** – Because of the altered state of senses and the physical reaction to the cannabinoids, you should always check your blood glucose level at regular intervals to ensure that you are in a safe range.
- **Keep Your Equipment Nearby** – Always keep your equipment in your usual spot so that you can easily access your blood testing equipment and medication when needed.
- **Never Medicate In Public** – Expect the unexpected. As with alcohol, you cannot expect to drive or work under influenced.
- **Bolus For "Munchies"** – You may get the "munchies" urge after administrating medical cannabis. If you are prone to eating habits, make sure to give yourself an insulin adjustment to compensate for the extra sugar and calories you will be eating.
- **Don't Forget "Edible" Carbs** – Edibles can contain large amounts of carbohydrates (that is why it tastes so good), fat, and calories. To mask the taste of cannabis, a "pot cookie" can contain much more sugar than your

usual cookies. So always remember to give yourself an adjusted dosage of insulin accordingly.

As with using any medication and altered sense substance, always be aware of your body's reaction and your surroundings. Remember that you should never feel pressured to try something that you do not feel safe or comfortable trying (sometimes a store sale may push a new product on you for profit and know very little about your medical conditions). The decision is up to you alone.

Over Consumption Of Marijuana

Consuming too much cannabis can be quite a very nasty experience. Anyone who has over-consumed marijuana edibles will tell you that not taking enough is far better than taking too much. Fortunately, marijuana is non-toxic to healthy human cells or organs, so you do not need to worry about dying from a cannabis overdose. However, that does not mean you should not worry about overconsumption. Taking in too much marijuana in one sitting can make you instantly regret the decision, and it can happen with any type of cannabis product if you are not careful.

Overconsumption is typically characterized by an increase in heart rate, accompanied by cold sweat, dryness of the mouth (also known as cottonmouth), extreme dizziness, similar to motion sickness, and/or feelings of paranoia or anxiety. It is very important to remember that these symptoms are only temporary and will usually dispel within fifteen minutes to an hour for smoked or vaporized cannabis flowers, slightly longer for concentrates, and anywhere from thirty minutes to two hours for infused products and edibles. If you know that you have overconsumed or you suspect you have overconsumed, try to stay calm and remember that the feeling is only temporary. Eating a bit of fatty food and drinking a lot of water can lessen the effect.

Afterward, lay or sit down, close your eyes, and try to relax. Keep your blood glucose testing kit close to you and check if necessary. If you are with someone, let them know that you have over-consume cannabis, and ask them to keep an eye on you just as a safety precaution. If your discomfort level becomes too unbearable that you think you need medical attention, ask someone to drive you to the emergency clinic or call 9-1-1 for emergency help assistance. Do NOT try to drive anywhere by yourself!

14. Conclusion

We hope that this short book has provided you with helpful information on how cannabis may be beneficial for pre-diabetic individuals, type 1 diabetic[29] or type 2 diabetic[30] and many other diseases. It is important to remember that, like medication, cannabis use should be limited to how much you need. If you have too little, you may not see any benefits in cannabis consumption. With the right amount, you can get the greatest benefits. But once you push over the limit, the benefits will plateau or even be harmful to your body in the long run. Before you consider whether medical marijuana may be a treatment option, please remember to check with your local regulations concerning the legality of using and obtaining cannabis as a medical treatment.

It is equally important to consult with your doctor[31] and obtain a prescription for using cannabis as your treatment. If you have any comments and/or experiences to share, please leave us a message and/or a comment in the review section of where you obtained a copy of this book. We would

---

[29] Anonymous. Type 1 Diabetes: An Overview. *The Diabetes Council.* https://www.thediabetescouncil.com/type-1-diabetes-an-overview/

[30] Anonymous. Type 2 Diabetes: An Overview. *The Diabetes Council.* https://www.thediabetescouncil.com/type-2-diabetes-an-overview/

[31] Anonymous. When To See Doctor. *The Diabetes Council.* https://www.thediabetescouncil.com/when-to-see-doctor/

absolutely love to hear from you, or please feel free to email us at MDumas@IncandescentInc.com

Definitions For Some Of The Components Of Cannabis

Tetrahydrocannabinol (THC) – THC is the most famous and abundant cannabinoid. THC is what causes the psychoactive "high" associated with cannabis use. THC also has analgesic and pain-killing properties.

Cannabidiol (CBD) – Another famous cannabinoid that has dramatically increased in popularity. CBD is a non-psychoactive component and is known for its ability to lessen anxiety, pain, and inflammation, but in recent years has become famous for its efficacy in reducing seizures.

Tetrahydrocannabinol Acid (THCA) – THCA is the forerunner to THC and several other cannabinoids. THCA is found in raw cannabis and converts to THC when heated. THCA has also been studied for its anti-inflammatory, anti-convulsant and nausea reducing properties.

Cannabidiolic Acid (CBDA) – CBDA is similar to THCA and is the forerunner to CBD in strains with high amounts of the cannabinoid (mostly hemp). It is akin to THCA in that it transforms to CBD when heated. CBDA is thought to contribute to hemp's anti-inflammatory properties due to its ability to hinder enzymes called COX-2, which is what the body produces after an injury. Research says that CBDA may help ease nausea and depression.

Cannabigerol (CBG) – CBG is a component that has recently grown in popularity because of its different potential benefits. Like CBD, CBG is non-psychoactive and is known for its antibacterial, blood pressure regulating and anti-inflammatory properties as well as being a sleep-aid.

Cannabinol (CBN) – CBN is slightly psychoactive and mostly used as a sedative that is dose-dependent, meaning that as the dose changes so does the effect. CBN is produced by the degrading of THC, it tends to show up in older cannabis. The amount of CBN produced is affected by how much exposure it receives to natural light – the more light, the higher the level of CBN. While CBN also has anti-inflammatory properties, it is currently being researched as a treatment for epilepsy, osteoporosis, cancer, bacterial infections, glaucoma, and nausea.

Cannabichromene (CBC) – CBC, like CBD is non-psychoactive and is also being researched as a possible pain reducer, tumor inhibitor and neuroprotectant *(an agent that serves to protect nerve cells against damage and/or degeneration)*. Studies are also showing CBC to be promising as a treatment for IBS (Irritable Bowel Syndrome), and Crohn's disease.

Tetrahydrocannabivarin (THCV) – THCV is very similar to THC and has only a small molecular difference. THCV is an exact opposite of its cousin THC in that it is known as an appetite suppressant rather than a stimulant. THCV is also praised for its potential in reducing anxiety, and also its ability to promote bone growth.

Cannabidivarin (CBDV) – CBDV, also like CBD, is non-psychoactive and differs very slightly in its molecular structure. CBDV is currently being researched as a possible treatment for epilepsy and has been known to be effective in decreasing nausea and inflammation. At the present, very little is known about this particular cannabinoid.

Terpenes – Terpenes are what give cannabis plants its aroma and flavor. Hundreds of terpenes are found in nature, but in cannabis there are eight main terpenes:

- Myrcene – The most prevalent terpene in cannabis, myrcene has a calming effect. It is also found in some varieties of mangoes and lemongrass. Myrcene is especially rich in classic strains such as Blue Dream and White Widow.
- Limonene – With hints of citrus fruits, limonene is known for its ability to relieve stress. This terpene is found in both sativa and indica-dominant strains, including Hindu Kush and Miracle Alien Cookies.
- Humulene – This terpene is also present in hops and is believed to have antibacterial and anti-inflammatory properties. High amounts of this terpene are found in strains such as Girl Scout Cookie and Headband.

- Terpinolene – This is the least common of the main terpenes, but popular and in great demand due to its near-psychedelic effects. Terpinolene is also found in tea tree essential oils and nutmeg. This herbal-esque terpene is found in strains such as Jack Herer and Dutch Treat.
- Linalool – Linalool is a popular ingredient in aromatherapy, its aroma is floral and fragrant. This terpene is also found in lavender and is known for its relaxing effects. Cannabis strains with higher amounts of linalool can be found in Zkittlez and Do-Si-Dos.
- Caryophyllene – This terpene is known for stress relief and for its ability to act as both a cannabinoid and a terpene. Caryophyllene has fragrant notes of spice and is present in cinnamon and black pepper. You can find this terpene in strains like Chem Dog and Sour Diesel.
- Pinene – Pinene, found in coniferous trees, smells somewhat like an evergreen forest; This terpene is uplifting. promotes memory retention, and is found in many sativa-dominant strains. It's also present in CBD-rich strains, such as Harlequin and Cannatonic.
- Ocimene – Ocimene is sweet but woodsy, and has shown efficacy as an anti-inflammatory and a potential treatment for diabetes. It can be found in strains like Amnesia Haze and Green Crack.

References Used

1. Ellis R.J., et al. (2009). Smoked medicinal Cannabis for neuropathic pain in HIV: a randomized, crossover clinical trial. Neuropsychopharmacol 2009; 34(3): 672-80.

2. Carter GT, Flanagan AM, Earleywine M, Abrams DI, Aggarwal SK, Grinspoon L. Cannabis in palliative medicine: improving care and reducing opioid-related morbidity. Am J Hosp Palliat Care 2011;28:297-303.

3. Penner, E.A. et al. (2013). The Impact of Marijuana Use on Glucose, Insulin, and Insulin Resistance among US Adults. The American Journal of Medicine, Volume 126 , Issue 7 , 583 – 589.

4. Ponz-Sarvise M, Nguewa PA, Pajares MJ, et al. Inhibitor of differentiation-1 as a novel prognostic factor in NSCLC patients with adenocarcinoma histology and its potential contribution to therapy resistance. Clin Cancer Res 2011;17:4155-66.

5. Soroceanu L, Murase R, Limbad C...Desprez PY, McAllister SD. Id-1 is a key transcriptional regulator of glioblastoma aggressiveness and a novel therapeutic target. Cancer Res 2013;73(5):1559-69. doi: 10.1158/0008-5472.CAN-12-1943. Epub 2012 Dec 13.

6. Velasco G, Sanchez C, Guzman M. Towards the use of cannabinoids as anti-tumor agents. Nature Reviews Cancer 12, 436-444 (June 2012) | doi:10.1038/nrc3247.

Website References

1. www.civilized.life/articles/marijuana-propaganda-movies/
2. https://medium.com/@liezeboshoff/the-story-of-charlottes-web-can-it-work-for-your-child-too-ecc4382e40b7
3. https://www.cnn.com/2013/08/07/health/charlotte-child-medical-marijuana/
4. https://www.forbes.com/sites/emilyearlenbaugh/2020/08/11/cannabis-shows-potential-to-help-and-harm-in-coronavirus-cases-experts-explain-why/#211602933ea6

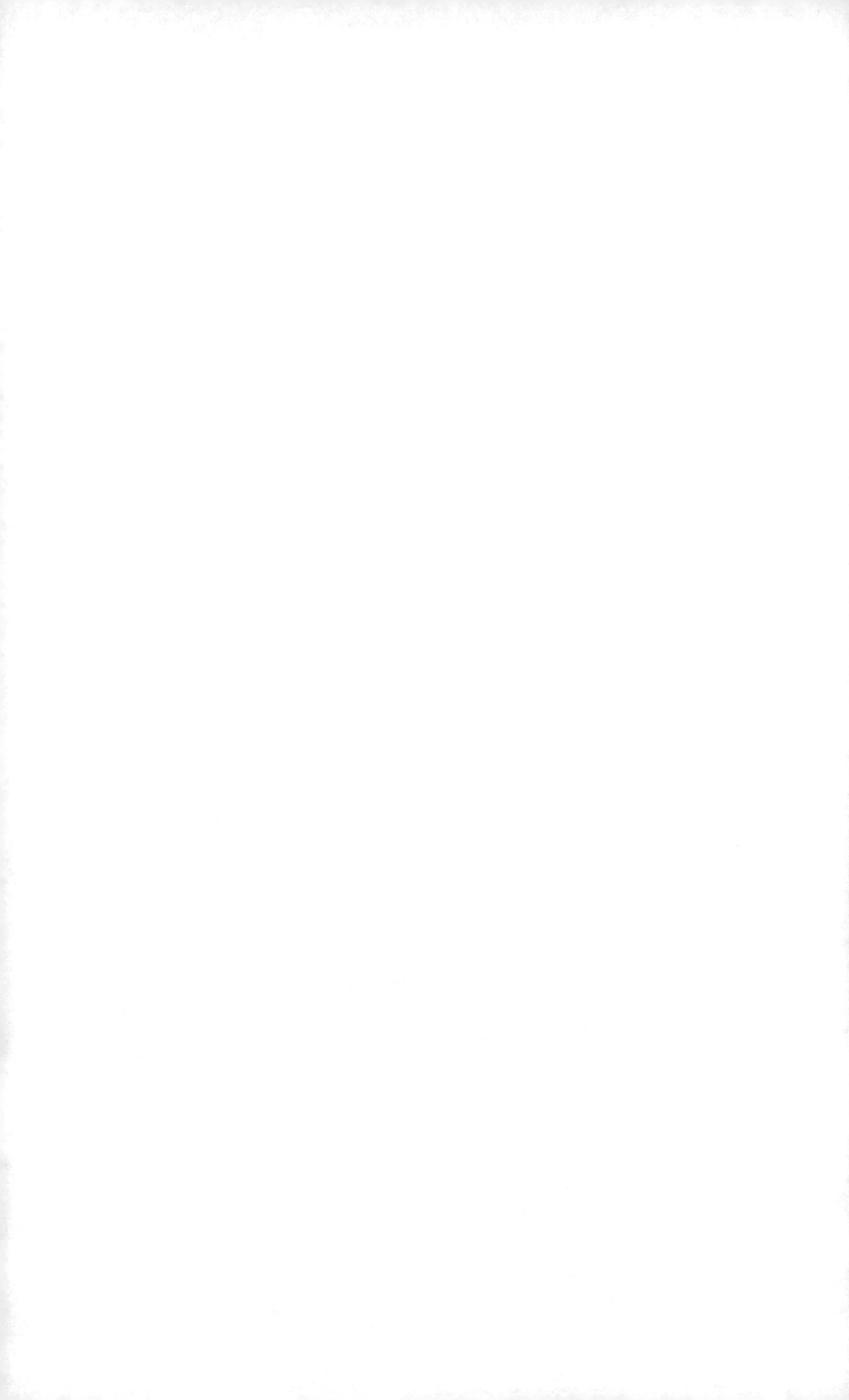

www.ingramcontent.com/pod-product-compliance
Ingram Content Group UK Ltd.
Pitfield, Milton Keynes, MK11 3LW, UK
UKHW021838270726
14058UKWH00002B/230

9 781915 206190